FATTY LIVER DIET COOKBOOK

2024

"1800 Days Quick & Healthy Low-Fat Recipes for Better Health and Longevity."

ERNEST G. MOORE

DISCLAIMER

Please note the information contain within this document is for educational and entertainment purpose only. All effort has been executed to present accurate, up to date, reliable, and complete information. No warranties of any kind are declared or implied. Readers acknowledge that the author is not engaged in the rendering of legal, financial, medical or professional advice. The content within this book has been derived from various sources. Please consult a licensed professional before attempting any techniques outlined in this book. By reading this document the reader agrees that under no circumstances is the author responsible for any losses, direct or indirect, that are incurred as a result of the use of the information contained within this document, including, but not limited to, errors, omissions, or inaccuracies.

TABLE OF CONTENTS

Introduction

Understanding fatty liver disease.

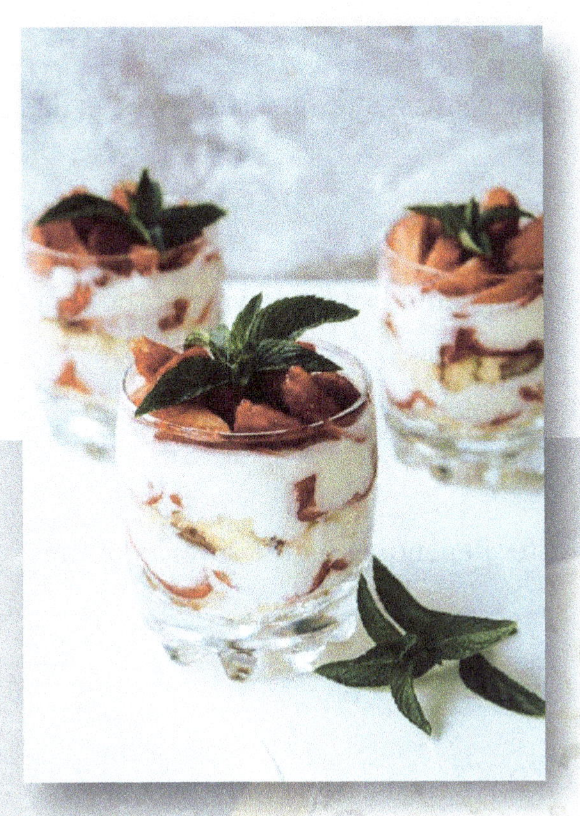

Fatty liver disease, also known as hepatic steatosis, is a disorder marked by the buildup of excess fat in liver cells. This disease may vary from moderate to severe, and it is often linked to other health problems, including obesity, diabetes, and metabolic syndrome. Understanding the underlying causes, symptoms, and possible consequences of fatty liver disease is critical for successful treatment and prevention.

THE CAUSES OF FATTY LIVER DISEASE ARE:

- ❖ **Nonalcoholic Fatty Liver Disease (NAFLD):** This is the most frequent kind of fatty liver disease, and it is not caused by excessive alcohol intake. NAFLD is significantly linked to obesity, insulin resistance, and metabolic syndrome. Genetics, food, and lifestyle choices all play an important role in its development.
- ❖ **Alcoholic Fatty Liver Disease (AFLD):** Excessive alcohol consumption over time causes AFLD. Alcohol is processed in the liver, and persistent alcohol consumption may result in liver cell fat buildup, inflammation, and, ultimately, liver damage.
- ❖ **Other Reasons:** Fatty liver disease may also be caused by certain medical circumstances, including fast weight loss, starvation, medicines, viral hepatitis, and genetic diseases.

SYMPTOMS OF FATTY LIVER DISEASE:

In its early stages, fatty liver disease may not produce any symptoms. However, as the illness progresses, people may experience:

Symptoms include fatigue and weakness.

Symptoms may include abdominal pain, swelling, and jaundice (yellowing of the skin and eyes).

Symptoms may include decreased appetite and unexplained weight loss.

Nausea or vomiting.

It's crucial to remember that symptoms might differ depending on the severity of the illness and any underlying diseases.

DIAGNOSIS AND EVALUATION:

Fatty liver disease is frequently detected during normal medical examinations or investigations for unrelated illnesses. Diagnostic tests may include:

- ❖ **Blood test:** Elevated liver enzymes, especially ALT and AST, may suggest liver inflammation or injury.
- ❖ **Imaging Studies:** Ultrasound, computed tomography (CT), and magnetic resonance imaging (MRI) scans may detect extra fat in the liver and determine its severity.
- ❖ **Liver biopsy:** In certain situations, a liver biopsy may be necessary to determine the amount of liver damage and rule out other liver illnesses.

COMPLICATIONS OF FATTY LIVER DISEASE:

If not addressed, fatty liver disease may progress to more serious disorders, such as:

- ❖ Non-alcoholic steatohepatitis (NASH) is a more severe variant of NAFLD that causes liver inflammation and damage.
- ❖ **Liver Fibrosis:** The accumulation of scar tissue in the liver may compromise function and progress to cirrhosis.

- ❖ **Cirrhosis:** advanced liver scarring that causes lifelong liver damage and dysfunction.
- ❖ **Liver Cancer:** Chronic inflammation and liver damage raise the chance of developing hepatocellular carcinoma.

TREATMENT AND MANAGEMENT:

The therapy and management of fatty liver disease are largely concerned with treating underlying risk factors and establishing a healthy lifestyle. This might include:

Weight reduction achieved by a healthy diet and regular exercise to minimize fat deposition in the liver.

managing underlying diseases, including obesity, diabetes, and high cholesterol.

Limiting or refraining from alcohol in the case of AFLD.

avoiding the use of hepatotoxic drugs and substances.

maintaining liver health with regular medical examinations and screening procedures.

Healthcare practitioners may offer drugs or therapies to treat specific fatty liver disease symptoms or problems.

CONCLUSION:

Fatty liver disease is a prevalent and potentially dangerous disorder that requires aggressive treatment and lifestyle changes. Individuals may avoid or lessen the effect of this condition on their liver health by learning its origins, symptoms, and possible consequences. Early discovery, thorough medical examination, and adherence to treatment guidelines are critical for maintaining liver function and general health.

The Role of Diet in Managing Fatty Liver

Diet is important in controlling fatty liver disease (FLD) because it directly affects liver fat buildup, inflammation, and overall liver function. A well-planned diet may help to decrease liver fat, slow disease development, and enhance liver function. Understanding the fundamentals of a liver-friendly diet and making the right food selections are critical components of FLD treatment.

KEY DIET GOALS

- ❖ **Weight management:** Excess body weight, especially visceral adiposity, is strongly associated with the onset and progression of fatty liver disease. Achieving and maintaining a healthy weight via calorie restriction and regular physical exercise is critical for controlling FLD.

- ❖ **Balanced Macronutrient Intake:** A balanced macronutrient intake—carbohydrates, proteins, and fats—is critical for liver function. Eat complex carbs, lean proteins, and healthy fats while reducing processed sugars and saturated fats.

- ❖ **Healthful Fats:** Incorporate healthy fat sources such as omega-3 fatty acids found in fatty fish (salmon, mackerel, and sardines), flaxseeds, chia seeds, and walnuts. These lipids are anti-inflammatory, which may help minimize liver fat buildup and inflammation.

- ❖ **Fiber-rich foods:** Fruits, vegetables, whole grains, legumes, and nuts are high in fiber, which promotes satiety, helps with weight control, and supports digestive health. Soluble fiber, in particular, helps manage blood sugar and cholesterol levels, both of which are crucial for those with fatty liver disease.

- ❖ **Limited sugar and refined carbs:** Excessive intake of added sugars and processed carbs may lead to insulin resistance, hepatic fat storage, and inflammation. Limit your consumption of sugary drinks, candies, pastries, and processed meals rich in refined grains.

❖ **Moderate Alcohol Consumption:** Individuals with alcoholic fatty liver disease (AFLD) should abstain from alcohol to avoid additional liver damage. Even modest alcohol use might worsen liver inflammation and increase liver fibrosis in FLD patients.

SPECIFIC DIETARY RECOMMENDATIONS:

❖ **The Mediterranean Diet:** The Mediterranean diet, which includes plenty of fruits and vegetables, whole grains, nuts, seeds, olive oil, and fish, has been linked to a lower incidence of fatty liver disease and better liver function.

❖ **Foods with a low glycemic index (GI):** Choose foods with a low glycemic index to help control blood sugar and prevent insulin resistance. Examples include non-starchy veggies, legumes, whole grains, and lean meats.

❖ **Foods that cleanse the liver:** Cruciferous vegetables (broccoli, Brussels sprouts, kale), garlic, onions, beets, artichokes, and turmeric are thought to be beneficial to liver health and detoxification processes.

❖ **Portion Control:** Pay attention to portion proportions. Using smaller plates, practicing mindful eating, and avoiding distractions during meals may all contribute to better portion management and attentive eating practices.

CONCLUSION:

A well-balanced, nutritious diet may help manage fatty liver disease by encouraging weight reduction, lowering liver fat deposition, and enhancing overall liver function. Individuals may promote liver health and reduce the risk of disease development by eating a diet rich in whole foods, healthy fats, fiber, and important nutrients. Combined with regular physical exercise and lifestyle changes, dietary treatments are the foundation of FLD management and contribute to long-term liver health and well-being.

Guidelines for Using This Cookbook

This cookbook is intended to assist patients with fatty liver disease (FLD) or those at risk of developing FLD with tasty and nutritious dishes that promote liver health and general well-being. To optimize the advantages of this cookbook and successfully manage FLD with dietary treatments, consider the following guidelines:

❖ **Be aware of your dietary goals:**
Each person may have different dietary objectives depending on their stage of fatty liver disease, general health, and personal preferences. Whether you want to lose weight, enhance liver function, regulate blood sugar levels, or decrease inflammation, knowing your individual dietary requirements can help you choose recipes and plan meals.

❖ **Refer to the serving sizes and nutritional information:**
Pay attention to the serving sizes and nutritional information given with each recipe. This information may help you make more educated decisions regarding portion size, calorie consumption, and nutritional content. Be aware of substances rich in added sugars, bad fats, or salt, and make substitutions or changes as appropriate.

❖ **Embrace Diversity and Balance:**
A well-balanced diet rich in nutrient-dense foods is vital for maintaining liver function and general well-being. Incorporate a variety of fruits, vegetables, whole grains, lean meats, and healthy fats into your meals to ensure you're getting enough nutrients while still having a full and tasty diet.

❖ **Customize Recipes to Meet Your Preferences and Dietary Restrictions:**
Feel free to modify recipes to suit your tastes, dietary constraints, or food allergies. Substitute foods, tweak spices, or change cooking techniques to meet your specific requirements and tastes while remaining true to the principles of a liver-friendly diet.

* **Practice portion control and mindful eating.**

  To maintain portion control, limit serving sizes and avoid large servings. Savor each mouthful, chew gently, and be aware of hunger and fullness signals. Eating thoughtfully may help you avoid overeating, improve your digestion, and have a better dining experience.

* **Engage in regular physical activity.**

  In addition to dietary adjustments, frequent physical exercise is critical for treating fatty liver disease and promoting overall health. Aim for at least 30 minutes of moderate-intensity activity most days of the week, such as brisk walking, cycling, swimming, or yoga, to help with weight loss, liver function, and inflammation reduction.

* **Track your progress and adjust as needed:**

  Keep track of your eating habits, physical activity levels, and any changes in symptoms or health outcomes that occur over time. Monitor your progress on a regular basis with your healthcare practitioner, and make adjustments to your dietary and lifestyle habits as required to reach your health goals and improve your fatty liver disease treatment.

* By adhering to these rules and incorporating the recipes and ideas presented in this cookbook into your daily routine, you can make proactive efforts to improve liver health, treat fatty liver disease, and enjoy a tasty and satisfying meal that feeds both body and spirit.

CHAPTER
1
BREAKFAST

INTRODUCTION TO BREAKFAST RECIPES

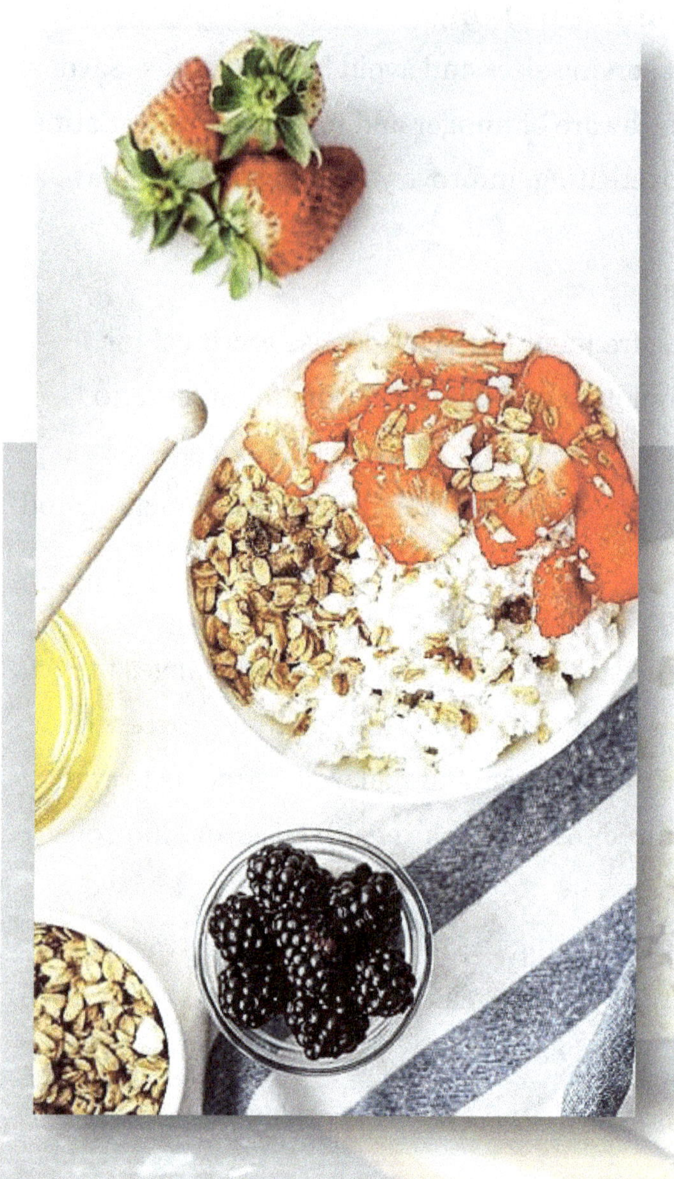

Start your day off right with a nourishing and satisfying breakfast! In this section of the cookbook, you'll find a variety of delicious breakfast recipes designed to support liver health and provide you with the energy and nutrients you need to kickstart your morning. From hearty bowls of oatmeal loaded with fresh berries to protein-packed omelettes and wholesome pancakes, there's something for everyone to enjoy. Whether you prefer sweet or savory flavors, these breakfast recipes are sure to delight your taste buds while helping you maintain a healthy lifestyle. So, rise and shine, and let's explore the wonderful world of breakfast delights!

Avocado Breakfast Bowl

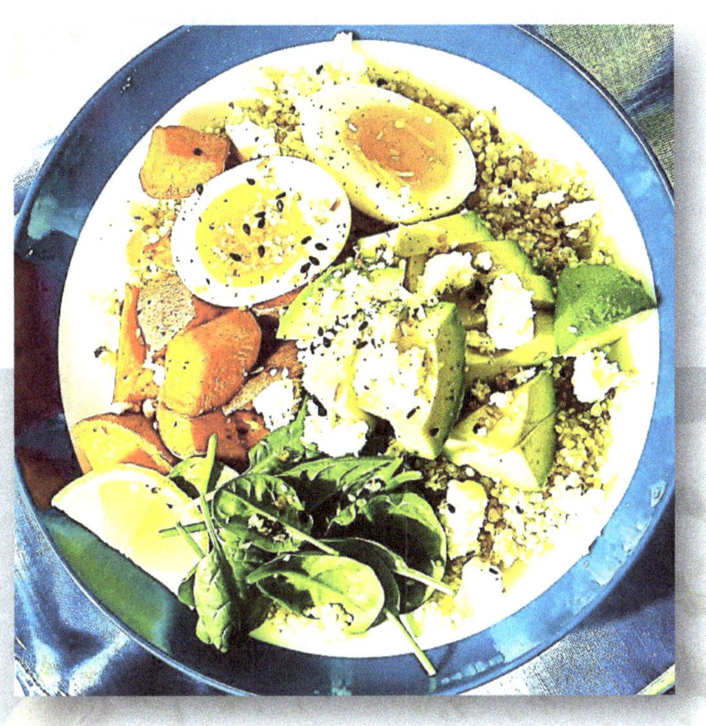

Prep time: 10 minutes.

Cooking time: none.

Serving Unit: One bowl.

Ingredients:

- One ripe avocado.
- 2 eggs
- To prepare, halve 1/4 cup cherry tomatoes and cube 1/4 cup cucumber.
- 2 tablespoons crumbled feta cheese and 1 tablespoon chopped fresh cilantro.
- Add salt and pepper to taste.
- Optional toppings include sliced radishes, microgreens, and spicy sauce.

Directions:

1. Slice the avocado in half and remove the pit. Scoop away some of the meat from each

side to provide a bigger cavity for the filling.

2. In a small bowl, mix the eggs until fully combined.

3. Heat a nonstick skillet over medium heat and add the beaten eggs. Cook the eggs, stirring occasionally, until they are scrambled and well cooked.

4. Place the scrambled eggs in the hollowed-out avocado halves.

5. Top the avocado halves with cherry tomatoes, cucumber, crumbled feta cheese, and fresh cilantro.

6. Add salt and pepper to taste.

7. Garnish with sliced radishes, micro greens, or a sprinkle of spicy sauce for more flavor and appearance.

8. Serve immediately and enjoy your healthy and tasty avocado breakfast bowl!

Nutrition Facts (per serving):

- Calories: 380
- Total fat: 29 grams.
- Saturated Fat: 7 grams
- Cholesterol: 390 mg.
- Sodium: 330 mg.
- Total carbs: 15g
- Dietary fiber: 9 grams
- Sugars: 2 grams
- Protein: 17 grams.

Tip:

- Select ripe avocados for optimal taste and texture. When pressed, they should give slightly under mild pressure.
- Top your avocado breakfast bowl with your preferred toppings and spices. Consider adding chopped bell peppers, onions, or jalapeños for more flavor and crunch.

- For a vegetarian version, skip the eggs and replace them with scrambled tofu or cooked quinoa.
- Preparing the materials ahead of time and assembling the avocado breakfast bowl immediately before serving will guarantee optimal freshness and quality.

Health benefits:

- **"Full of Healthy Fats"** Avocados are high in heart-healthy monounsaturated fats, which may help decrease bad cholesterol and cut the risk of heart disease.
- Avocados are high in dietary fiber, which promotes digestive health while also providing a sense of fullness and contentment.
- **Protein Power:** Eggs are a complete protein source that contains all nine essential amino acids required for muscle repair and development.
- **Nutrient-Rich:** The fresh veggies in this breakfast bowl are high in vitamins, minerals, and antioxidants, all of which are vital for general health and wellness.
- **Balanced Meal:** This avocado breakfast bowl, which includes healthy fats, protein, and fiber-rich veggies, provides a balanced and nutritious start to the day, helping to regulate blood sugar levels and avoid mid-morning energy dumps.

Enjoy the creamy deliciousness of avocado with healthful ingredients in this nutrient-dense breakfast dish that will energize your body while tantalizing your taste buds!

Oatmeal with Berries

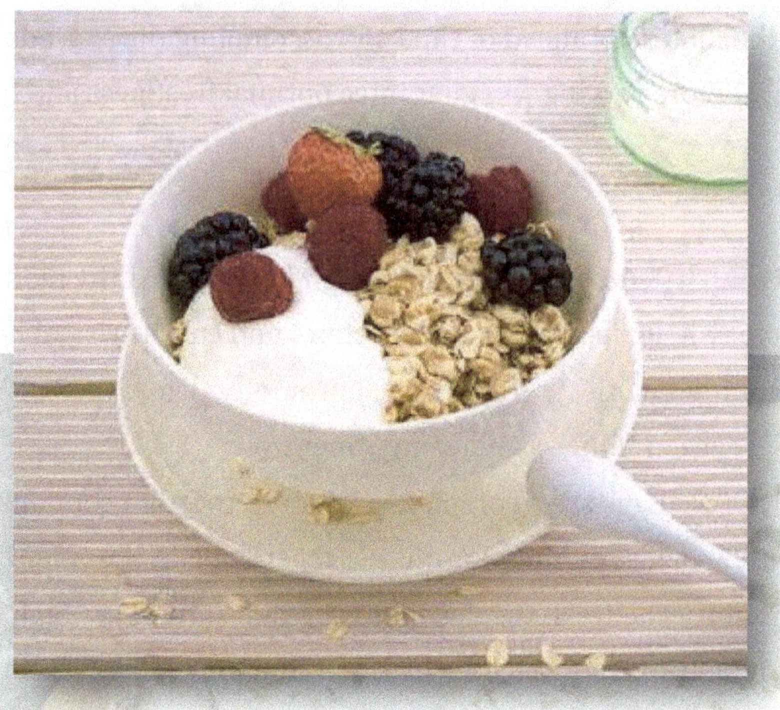

Prep Time: 5 minutes

Cooking Time: 10 minutes.

Serving Unit: One bowl.

Ingredients:

- 1/2 cup rolled oats and 1 cup water or milk (dairy or plant-based).
- 1/2 cup mixed berries (strawberries, blueberries, and raspberries)
- 1 tablespoon of honey or maple syrup.
- 1 tablespoon of chopped nuts (almonds, walnuts, or pecans).
- A pinch of cinnamon (optional).
- A pinch of salt.

Directions:

1. Heat the water or milk in a small saucepan over medium heat until it boils.

2. Stir in the rolled oats and turn the heat down to low. Simmer, stirring regularly, for approximately 5-7 minutes, or until the oats reach your preferred consistency.

3. Once the oats are cooked, take the skillet off the heat and let it rest for a minute to thicken.

4. Transfer the cooked oats to a serving dish.

5. Top the oats with mixed berries, honey or maple syrup, and chopped nuts.

6. Optional: Add a sprinkle of cinnamon for added taste.

7. Gently stir together all of the ingredients.

8. Serve warm and enjoy your delicious and healthy oatmeal with berries!

Nutrition Facts (per serving):

- Calories: 280
- Total fat: 6 grams.
- Saturated fat: 1g
- Cholesterol: 0 mg.
- Sodium: 70 mg.
- Total Carbohydrates: 50 grams
- Dietary fiber: 8 grams
- Sugars: 15 grams
- Protein: 9 grams.

Tip:

- Use old-fashioned rolled oats for optimal texture and taste. Avoid quick oats, since they may include additional sugars and lack the same substantial feel.
- Top your oats with your favorite ingredients, such as sliced bananas, chopped apples, dried fruits, or shredded coconut.
- Cook the oats in milk instead of water for a creamier consistency.
- Make a big pot of oats and keep the leftovers in the fridge for quick and easy breakfasts throughout the week. Simply reheat in the microwave or on the stovetop, and serve with fresh toppings.

Health Benefits:

- **Whole Grain Goodness:** Oats are high in soluble fiber, which helps decrease cholesterol and improve heart health. They also include complex carbs, which provide long-term energy.

- **Antioxidant Power:** Berries are high in antioxidants, such as vitamin C and flavonoids, which protect cells from free radical damage and boost immunological function.

- **Heart-Healthy Fats:** Nuts include heart-healthy unsaturated fats, as well as protein and fiber, which may help you feel full and content.

- **Natural Sweetness:** Honey and maple syrup add natural sweetness to oats, eliminating the need for refined sweeteners and providing a healthy option for satisfying your sweet craving.

- **Nutrient-Rich:** This oatmeal with berries is both tasty and nutrient-dense, including critical vitamins, minerals, and antioxidants that promote overall health and wellness.

Indulge in the soothing warmth of oats combined with the natural sweetness of berries for a balanced and enjoyable breakfast that will fuel your body while also pleasing your palate!

Spinach and Feta Omelet

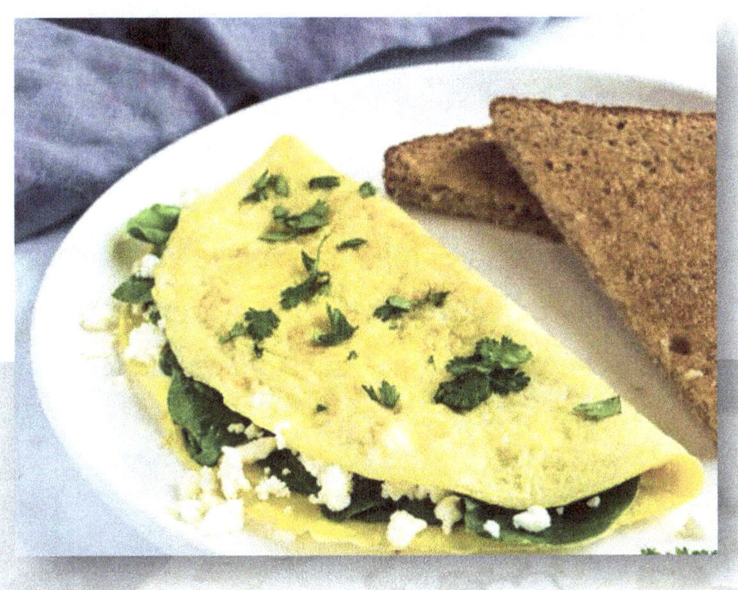

Prep Time: 5 minutes

Cooking Time: 5 minutes.

Serving Unit: One omelette.

Ingredients:

- Two big eggs.
- 1/2 cup of fresh spinach leaves chopped
- Ingredients: 1/4 cup crumbled feta cheese, 1 tablespoon olive oil.
- Season to taste with salt and pepper.
- Add optional toppings such as diced tomatoes, mushrooms, and bell peppers.

Directions:

1. In a small bowl, whisk the eggs until completely combined. To taste, season with salt and pepper.

2. Warm the olive oil in a nonstick skillet over medium heat.

3. Add the chopped spinach to the pan and cook for 1-2 minutes, until wilted.

4. Pour the beaten eggs over the spinach in the pan and distribute them evenly.

5. Cook the eggs without stirring for 2-3 minutes, or until the bottom is set and the sides begin to lift off the pan.

6. Distribute the crumbled feta cheese equally over one side of the omelet.

7. Using a spatula, delicately fold the remaining half of the omelette over the filling to make a half-moon shape.

8. Cook for a further 1-2 minutes, or until the cheese melts and the eggs are fully cooked.

9. Transfer the omelette to a platter and decorate with any preferred toppings.

10. Serve hot and enjoy your delicious and healthy spinach and feta omelette!

Nutrition Facts (per serving)

- Calories: 280
- Total fat: 21 grams.
- Saturated Fat: 7 grams
- Cholesterol: 385 mg.
- Sodium: 510 mg.
- Total carbs: 3 g.
- Dietary fiber: 1 gram
- Sugar: 1g.
- 19 grams of protein.

Tip:

- Use fresh spinach for optimal taste and texture. You may also use other leafy greens, like kale or Swiss chard.
- Crumble the feta cheese evenly over the omelette to ensure that every mouthful is full of great taste.
- For added taste and nutrients, top your omelette with diced tomatoes, sliced mushrooms, or chopped bell peppers.
- For a dairy-free version, replace the feta cheese with a dairy-free cheese or eliminate it entirely and add more veggies for taste and texture.

Health Benefits:

- **Protein Power:** Eggs include high-quality protein with all nine essential amino acids for muscle repair and development.
- **Leafy Greens:** Spinach is high in vitamins A, C, K, folate, iron, and magnesium. It is also low in calories and carbs, making it a good option for supplementing your diet without adding unnecessary calories.
- **Calcium Boost:** Feta cheese contains calcium, which is necessary for healthy bones and teeth.
- **Heart-Healthy Fats:** Olive oil contains monounsaturated fats, which may decrease inflammation and cut the risk of heart disease.
- **Minimal carbohydrate option:** This spinach and feta omelette is minimal in carbs and sugar, making it an ideal alternative for those on a low-carb or ketogenic diet.

Enjoy the savory richness of spinach and feta cheese wrapped in fluffy eggs for a tasty and healthy breakfast that will power your day and keep you full until lunch!

Whole-grain pancakes with fresh fruit

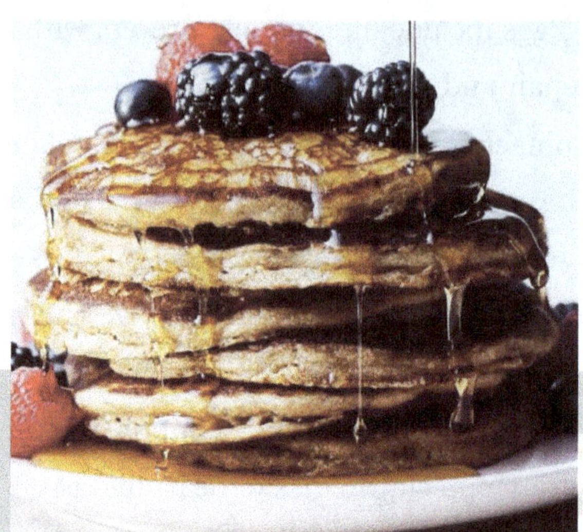

Prep Time: 10 minutes

Cooking Time: 10 minutes.

Serving Unit: One serving (about 2-3 pancakes).

Ingredients:

- Use 1 cup whole wheat flour and 1 tablespoon baking powder.
- 1 tablespoon of honey or maple syrup.
- 1 egg, 1 cup milk (dairy or vegan)
- One tablespoon of melted butter or oil.
- 1/2 teaspoon of vanilla essence.
- Add a pinch of salt.
- Top with fresh fruit, such as sliced strawberries, blueberries, or bananas.
- Maple syrup or honey to drizzle.

Directions:

1. In a large mixing basin, blend the whole wheat flour, baking powder, and salt until well incorporated.

2. In a separate dish, combine the egg, milk, melted butter or oil, honey or maple syrup,

and vanilla extract. Whisk until smooth.

3. Add the wet ingredients to the dry ones and whisk just until incorporated. Be cautious not to overmix; a few lumps are OK.

4. Heat a nonstick pan or griddle over medium heat and gently coat with butter or oil.

5. For each pancake, pour about 1/4 cup batter into the griddle. Cook until bubbles appear on the pancake's surface and the edges begin to set, approximately 2–3 minutes.

6. Flip the pancakes and heat for another 1-2 minutes, until golden brown and cooked through.

7. Repeat with the remaining batter, adding extra butter or oil to the pan if necessary.

8. Place the pancakes on a platter and top with the fresh fruit.

9. Optional: Drizzle with maple syrup or honey.

10. Enjoy your nutritious and tasty whole-grain pancakes with fresh fruit!

Nutrition Information (per serving, excluding toppings):

- Calorie: 250
- Total fat: 6 grams.
- Saturated fat: 3 g
- Cholesterol: 55 mg.
- Sodium: 400 mg.
- Total carbs: 40g.
- Dietary fiber: 5 grams
- Sugars: 7 grams
- Protein: 10 grams.

Tips:

- Choose whole wheat flour for more fiber and nutrients compared to refined white flour.
- To adjust the sweetness of the pancakes, add more or less honey or maple syrup to your liking.
- For added taste, sprinkle a bit of cinnamon or nutmeg into the batter.

- Place the pancakes on a baking sheet in a preheated oven at 200°F (95°C) to keep them warm while the rest of the batch cooks.
- Be creative with your toppings! Aside from fresh fruit, you may add nuts, seeds, yogurt, or a dab of nut butter to boost taste and nutrients.

Health benefits:

- **Whole Grains:** Whole wheat flour contains fiber, vitamins, and minerals that are removed from refined white flour, boosting digestive health and delivering lasting energy.
- **Protein:** Eggs are high in protein, which is required for muscle repair and development, as well as to maintain satiety and blood sugar levels.
  Fruit Power: Fresh fruit toppings add natural sweetness, vitamins, minerals, and antioxidants to the pancakes, which promotes general health and well-being.
- **Heart Health:** Whole-grain pancakes are low in saturated fat and cholesterol, making them a heart-healthy breakfast option when cooked with a minimum of additional fats and sweets.
- **Balanced Nutrition:** This breakfast choice has a variety of carbs, protein, and healthy fats, which will keep you feeling full and energetic throughout the morning.

Indulge in the healthy deliciousness of whole grain pancakes topped with fresh fruit for a nutritious and gratifying meal that will fuel your body while also pleasing your taste buds!

Greek Yogurt Parfait with Honey and Almonds

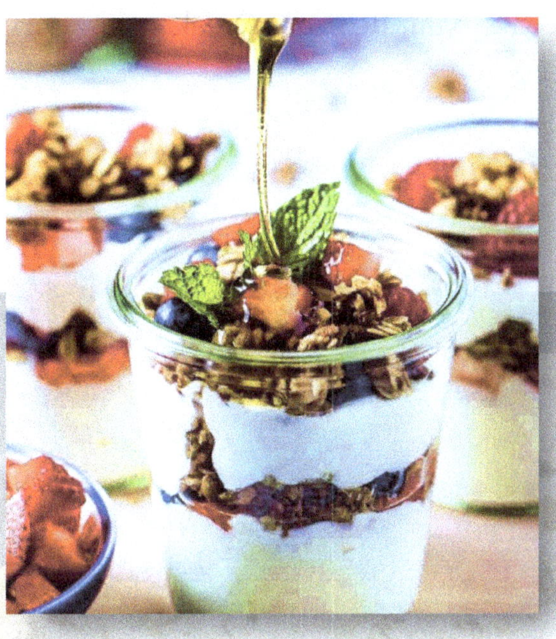

Prepare Time: 5 minutes

Cooking Time: 5 minutes

Serving Unit: One parfait.

Ingredients:

- 1/2 cup Greek yogurt, plain or flavored
- Ingredients: 1 tablespoon honey; 2 tablespoons chopped almonds.
- 1/4 cup fresh berries (strawberries, blueberries, or raspberries).
- 1 tablespoon granola (optional for extra crunch)

Directions:

1. In a small dish or glass, place half of the Greek yogurt.

2. Drizzle the yogurt with half the honey.

3. Combine half of the chopped almonds with the honey.

4. Arrange half of the fresh berries on top of the almonds.

5. Repeat layering with the remaining Greek yogurt, honey, almonds, and berries.

6. If preferred, add granola to the last layer for extra crunch and texture.

7. Serve immediately, and enjoy your delicious Greek yogurt parfait with honey and nuts.

Nutrition Facts (per serving):

- Calorie: 250
- Total fat: 10 grams
- Saturated Fat: 1.5 grams
- Cholesterol: 10 mg.
- Sodium: 40 mg.
- Total carbs: 25g
- Dietary Fiber: 3 grams
- Sugars: 18 grams
- Protein: 15 grams.

Tips:

- For a tart taste, use plain Greek yogurt. For extra sweetness, use flavored Greek yogurt (e.g., vanilla or honey).
  For a vegan version, use maple syrup or agave nectar instead of honey.
- Toast the sliced almonds briefly in a dry pan over medium heat to improve their taste and crunch.
- For more variety and nutrition, top your parfait with your favorite fruits, nuts, or seeds.
- Prepare the parfait ahead of time and refrigerate until ready to serve. To keep the granola crunchy, add it just before serving.

Health benefits:

- **Protein Boost:** Greek yogurt has a high concentration of protein, which promotes muscle development, repair, and satiety, making it an ideal breakfast or snack option.
- **Healthy Fats:** Almonds include heart-healthy monounsaturated fats and omega-3 fatty acids, which help to decrease inflammation and promote cardiovascular health.
- **Antioxidant Power:** Fresh berries are high in antioxidants, such as vitamin C and flavonoids, which protect cells from free radical damage and boost immunological function.
- **Digestive Health:** Greek yogurt also contains probiotics, which are good bacteria that improve gut health and digestion by maintaining a healthy balance of microorganisms in the digestive system.
- **Energy Boost:** This Greek yogurt parfait has a combination of carbs, protein, and healthy fats, making it a nutritious and stimulating breakfast or snack choice to start your day.

Enjoy the creamy deliciousness of Greek yogurt topped with sweet honey, crunchy almonds, and juicy berries for a delightful and healthy parfait that will both please your taste buds and feed your body!

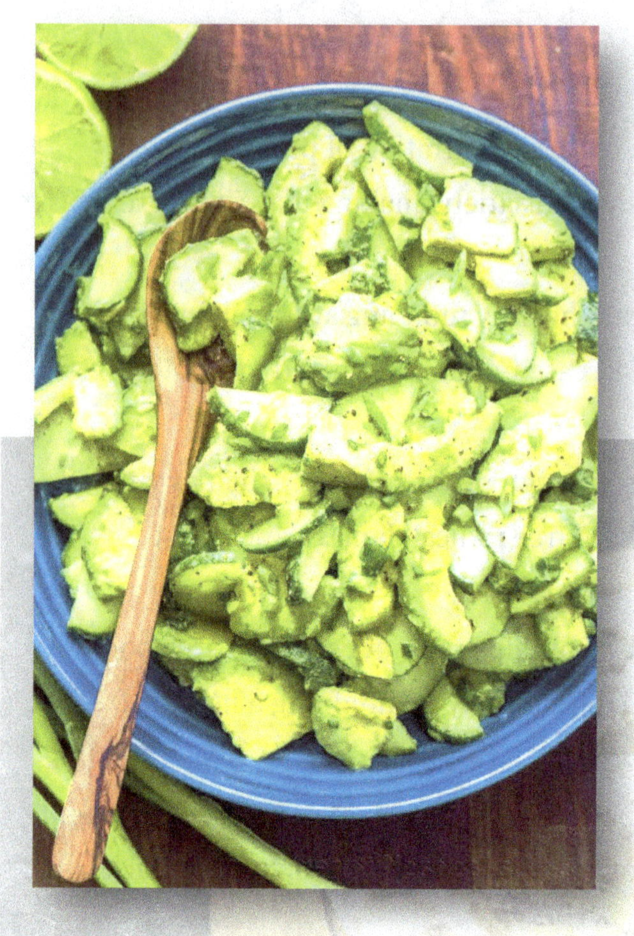

CHAPTER 2

APPETIZERS AND SNACKS

This part of the cookbook has a delectable selection of appetizers and nibbles meant to tickle your taste buds and keep hunger at bay in between meals. These dishes range from crisp vegetable sticks with creamy hummus to tasty quinoa-filled mushrooms and vivid cucumber-apple salsa, making them ideal for entertaining guests or fulfilling your own wants for something delicious and filling. Whether you're searching for a light and healthy snack or a crowd-pleasing appetizer, this wide assortment of dishes will provide inspiration and culinary enjoyment. So prepare to go on a delectable adventure through the world of appetizers and snacks that will take your munching experience to new heights!

Baked Sweet Potato Fries

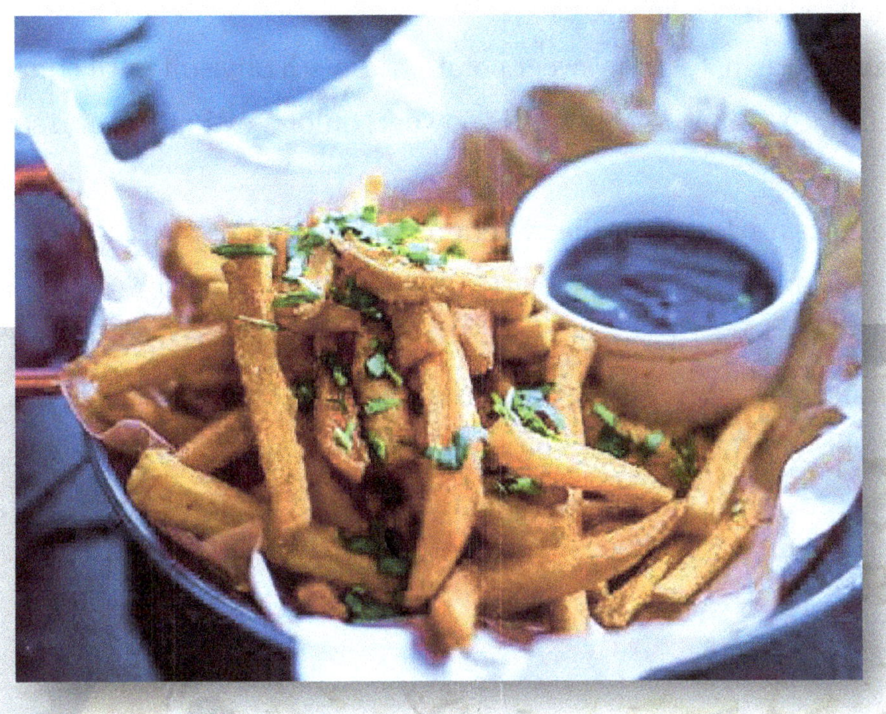

Prep Time: 10 minutes

Cooking Time: 25 minutes.

Serving Size: 2-4 servings

Ingredients:

- 2 medium sweet potatoes peeled and chopped into fries two teaspoons of olive oil.
- One teaspoon of paprika.
- One-half teaspoon garlic powder
- One-half teaspoon onion powder
- One-half teaspoon cumin
- Season to taste with salt and pepper.
- Garnish with fresh herbs (e.g., parsley, cilantro).

Directions:

1. Preheat the oven to 425°F (220°C) and prepare a baking sheet with parchment paper or aluminum foil for easy clean-up.

2. In a large mixing basin, toss the sweet potato fries with olive oil until equally coated.

3. In a small bowl, combine paprika, garlic powder, onion powder, cumin, salt, and pepper.

4. Sprinkle the spice mixture over the sweet potato fries and toss to coat.

5. Arrange the seasoned sweet potato fries in a single layer on the prepared baking sheet, leaving enough space between them to achieve crispiness.

6. Bake in a preheated oven for 20–25 minutes, turning halfway through, or until the fries are golden brown and crispy on the surface but soft within.

7. Remove from the oven and let it cool slightly before serving.

8. Garnish with fresh herbs, if preferred, and serve hot with your favorite dip.

Nutrition Facts (per serving):

- Calorie: 150
- Total fat: 7 grams.
- Saturated fat: 1g
- Cholesterol: 0 mg.
- Sodium: 150 mg.
- Total carbs: 21g.
- Dietary fiber: 4 grams
- Sugars: 6 grams
- Protein: 2 grams.

Tips

- To get crispy sweet potato fries, chop them into consistent sizes and spread them out in a single layer on a baking pan. Avoid overcrowding.
- Feel free to adjust the seasoning to your liking. For more heat, sprinkle with cayenne pepper or use your preferred seasoning combination.

- To get additional crispiness, soak the chopped sweet potato fries in cold water for 30 minutes before patting dry and tossing with olive oil and seasonings.
- Dip the baked sweet potato fries in a variety of condiments, such as ketchup, barbecue sauce, aioli, or sriracha mayo, for more taste and delight.
- Sweet potato fries may be refrigerated in an airtight container for up to two days. Place them on a baking sheet and reheat in a preheated oven at 350°F (175°C) for 5–10 minutes, or until warm and crispy.

Health and B enefits

- Sweet potatoes are nutrient-dense and high in vitamins, minerals, and antioxidants such as vitamin A, C, potassium, and beta-carotene, which promote general health.
- **Fiber Power:** Sweet potatoes are high in dietary fiber, which helps with digestion, satiety, and blood sugar regulation.
- **Heart Health:** Olive oil contains monounsaturated fats, which have been found to benefit heart health by lowering bad cholesterol and decreasing the risk of cardiovascular disease.
- **Antioxidant Properties:** The spices in the seasoning blend, such as paprika and cumin, include antioxidants that help protect cells from free radical damage and promote immunological function.
- **Lower calorie content:** Baking sweet potato fries rather than frying them lowers their total calorie content and harmful fats, giving them a healthier alternative to regular fries without compromising taste or texture.

Enjoy the irresistible mix of crispy baked sweet potato fries, perfectly seasoned with fragrant spices, olive oil, and a pinch of salt. These guilt-free fries are a tasty and healthy snack or side dish that will fulfill your cravings and keep you wanting more!

Hummus and Crudité

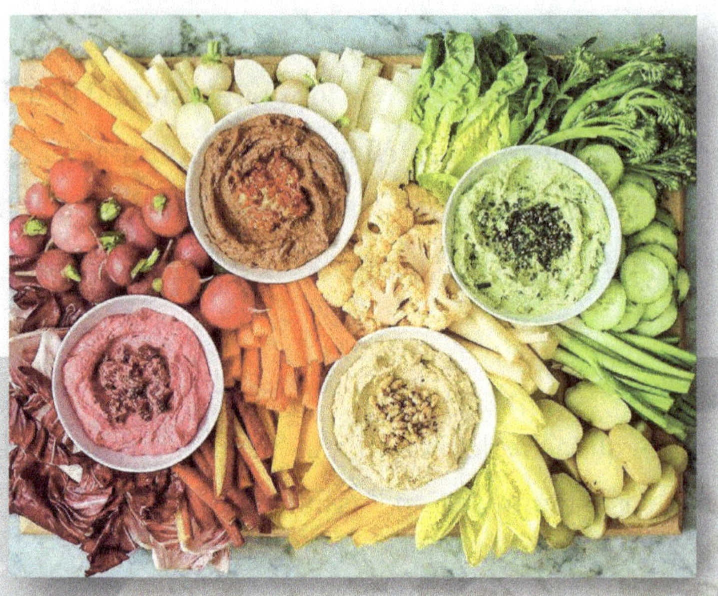

Prep Time: 10 min.

Serving Unit: 4 serves

Ingredients:

- Drain and rinse one can (15 ounces) of chickpeas. Mince two cloves of garlic.
- 3 tablespoons tahini (sesame paste) and 3 tablespoons lemon juice.
- Two teaspoons of olive oil.
- 1/2 teaspoon ground cumin.
- Season with salt and pepper to taste. Add crudité (washed and chopped fresh veggies, including carrots, cucumbers, bell peppers, cherry tomatoes, and celery).
- Optional garnish: chopped fresh parsley, a drizzle of olive oil, and a sprinkle of paprika.

Directions:

1. In a food processor, mix together the chickpeas, garlic, tahini, lemon juice, olive oil, ground cumin, salt, and pepper.

2. Blend the ingredients until smooth and creamy, scraping down the sides of the bowl

as necessary. If the hummus is too thick, add a tablespoon of water at a time until you get the ideal consistency.

3. Taste the hummus and season as needed, adding extra lemon juice, salt, or cumin to taste.

4. Place the hummus in a serving dish and top with chopped fresh parsley, olive oil, and paprika, if preferred.

5. Place the crudité sticks or bite-sized pieces around the bowl of hummus for dipping.

6. Serve immediately, and enjoy your delicious and healthy hummus with crudités!

Nutrition Information (per serving, excluding crudités):

- Calories: 160.
- Total fat: 10 grams.
- Saturated Fat: 1.5 grams
- Cholesterol: 0 mg.
- Sodium: 170 mg.
- Total carbs: 14g.
- Dietary fiber: 3 grams
- Sugar: 1g.
- Protein: 5 grams.

Tips

- To add flavor and diversity to your hummus, try adding roasted red peppers, sun-dried tomatoes, fresh herbs (e.g., parsley or cilantro), or za'atar spice mix.
  To get a smoother hummus, peel the chickpeas before mixing by gently pressing them between your fingers.
- Make a big batch of hummus and refrigerate it in an airtight container for up to a week. Serve as a nutritious snack, spread on sandwiches or wraps, or dip with crackers or pita bread.
- To add diversity and color to your plate, try dipping several kinds of crudité, such as blanched asparagus spears, radishes, sugar snap peas, or broccoli florets.

- To keep sliced veggies from drying out, place them in a jar of cold water in the refrigerator until ready to serve. Drain them well before placing them on the serving plate.

Health benefits:

- **Protein and Fiber-Rich:** Chickpeas are high in plant-based protein and dietary fiber, which aid in satiety, blood sugar regulation, and digestive health.
- **Heart-Healthy Fats:** Tahini and olive oil include heart-healthy monounsaturated fats and omega-3 fatty acids, which help to decrease inflammation and lessen the risk of heart disease.
- **Antioxidant Power:** Garlic, lemon juice, and olive oil are high in antioxidants, which help protect cells from free radical damage and maintain immunological function.
- **Vitamins and Minerals:** Chickpeas include a variety of vitamins and minerals, including vitamin K, folate, iron, magnesium, and zinc, all of which are necessary for optimal health.
- **Low Calorie:** Hummus is a nutrient-dense, low-calorie dish that is ideal for snacking or dipping without adding unnecessary calories or bad fats.

Dip into the creamy richness of homemade hummus, combined with vivid and crunchy crudité, for a filling and healthy snack that will keep you going throughout the day!

Cucumber and Avocado Salsa

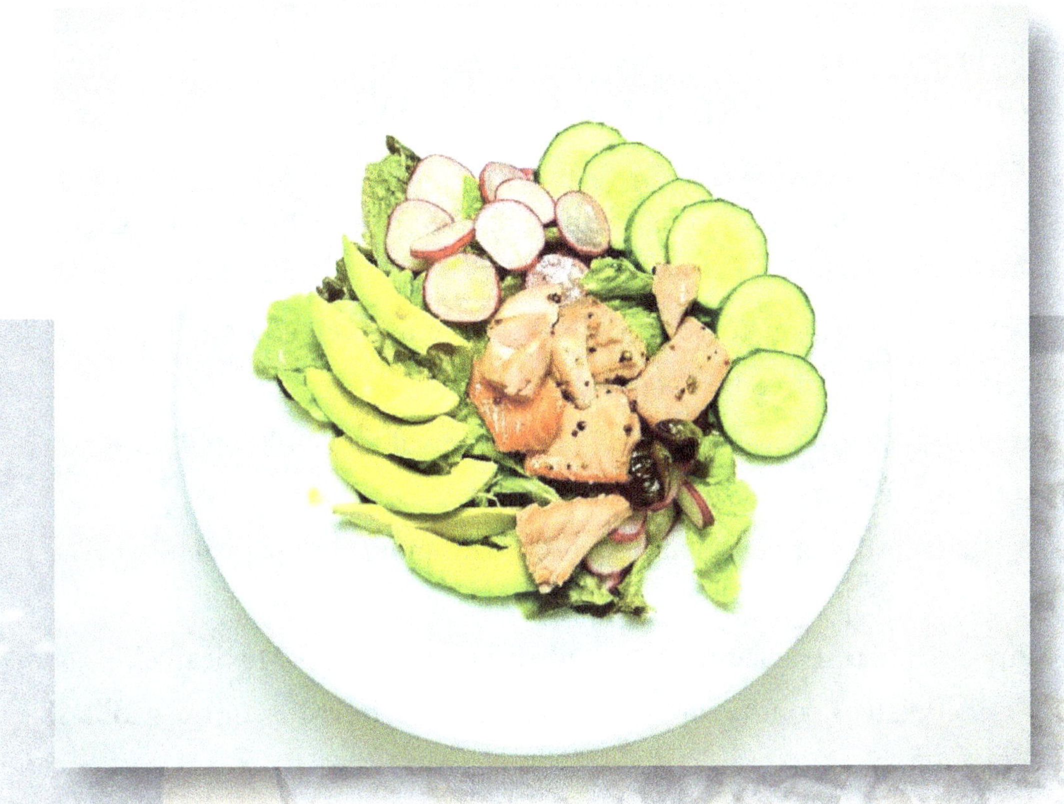

Prep Time: 10 min.

Serving Unit: 4 serves

Ingredients:

- To prepare, dice 1 big cucumber, 1 ripe avocado, 1/2 finely chopped red onion, and 1 seeded and finely sliced jalapeño pepper.
- 1/4 cup fresh cilantro, chopped
- 2 teaspoons of lime juice.
- One tablespoon of olive oil.
- Season to taste with salt and pepper.
- Optional ingredients include chopped tomatoes, corn kernels, black beans, and diced bell peppers.

Directions:

1. In a large mixing bowl, add diced cucumber, avocado, red onion, jalapeño pepper, and cilantro.

2. Drizzle the lime juice and olive oil over the items in the bowl.

3. Season with salt and pepper to taste, and then gently toss to mix all of the ingredients until equally coated.

4. Taste the salsa and adjust seasoning as needed, adding more lime juice, salt, or pepper to taste.

5. Optional additions for taste, texture, and color include chopped tomatoes, corn kernels, black beans, and diced bell peppers.

6. Serve the cucumber-avocado salsa right away, or cover and chill for at least 30 minutes to enable the flavors to combine before serving.

7. Before serving, stir the salsa well and sprinkle with more chopped cilantro, if preferred.

8. Serve your cool and tasty cucumber avocado salsa as a dip for Mexican chips, a topping for grilled fish or poultry, or a side dish for tacos, burritos, or quesadillas!

Nutrition Facts (per serving):

- Calories: 120.
- Total fat: 9 grams.
- Saturated Fat: 1.5 grams
- Cholesterol: 0 mg.
- Sodium: 10 mg.
- Total carbs: 10g
- Dietary fiber: 5 grams
- Sugars: 2 grams
- Two grams of protein.

Tip:

- Use ripe avocados for optimal taste and texture. When pressed, they should give slightly under mild pressure.
- Customize the salsa based on your flavor preferences and the seasonal availability of components. Feel free to add or swap ingredients according to what you have on hand.
- To make a milder salsa, remove the seeds and membranes from jalapeño peppers before chopping. If you want a hotter salsa, leave the seeds and membranes intact or add a sprinkle of cayenne pepper.
- Prepare the salsa ahead of time and refrigerate it in an airtight jar for up to 24 hours. The flavors will continue to develop with time, making it even more wonderful.
- Cucumber avocado salsa is a healthy and delicious appetizer, snack, or side dish for summer parties, picnics, and barbecues. It will undoubtedly be popular with both friends and family!

Health benefits:

- **Heart-Healthy Fats:** Avocado and olive oil include monounsaturated fats, which may help decrease bad cholesterol and lessen the risk of heart disease.
- **Hydration:** Cucumbers have a high water content, which helps to keep you hydrated and promotes good skin and digestion.
- **Vitamins and minerals:** Avocados and cucumbers are high in vitamins, minerals, and antioxidants, including vitamin C, vitamin K, potassium, and folate, which promote general health and well-being.
- **Digestive Health:** Cucumbers include dietary fiber, which improves digestion, increases satiety, and regulates bowel motions.
- **Low Calorie:** This cucumber avocado salsa has few calories and no additional sweets or bad fats, making it a healthy and guilt-free complement to your diet.

Quinoa-stuffed mushroom

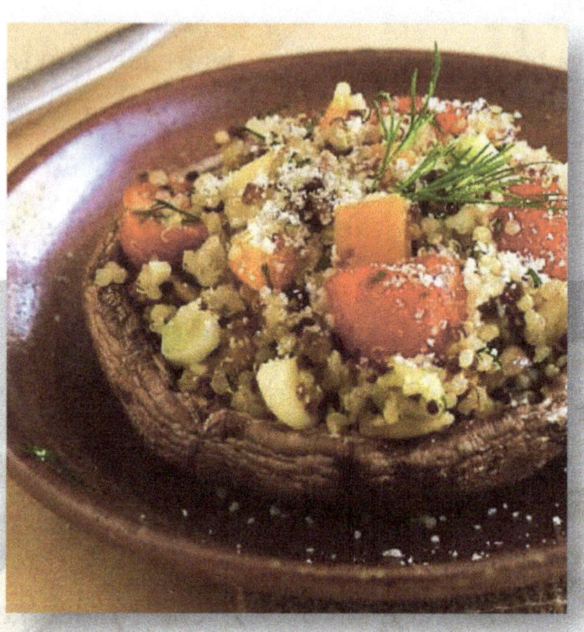

Preparation time: 15 minutes

Cooking time: 25 minutes

Total time: 40 minutes

Serving size: 4

Nutritional Data (Per Serving):

- Calories: 200 kcal.
- Protein: 8 grams.
- Fat: 10g
- Carbohydrate: 20 grams
- Fiber: 4 grams.
- Sugar: 2 grams.
- Sodium: 300 mg.

Ingredients:

- 16 big mushrooms (stems removed), 1 cup cooked quinoa, 1/2 cup chopped onion, and 1/2 cup diced bell pepper (of any color).
- 2 garlic cloves, minced
- Combine 1/4 cup grated Parmesan cheese;
- 1/4 cup chopped fresh parsley, and 2 tablespoons olive oil.
- Add salt and pepper to taste.

Directions:

1. Preheat the oven to 375°F (190°C).
2. Arrange the mushrooms on a baking sheet, gills facing up.
3. In a pan, heat 1 tablespoon of olive oil over medium heat. Combine the chopped onion, bell pepper, and garlic. Cook for about 5 minutes, or until softened.
4. In a mixing dish, mix together the cooked quinoa, sautéed veggies, Parmesan cheese, parsley, salt, and pepper. Mix thoroughly.
5. Spoon the quinoa mixture into each mushroom cap, gently pushing down to compress it in.
6. Drizzle the packed mushrooms with the remaining olive oil.
7. Bake in the preheated oven for 20–25 minutes, or until the mushrooms are soft and the filling is golden brown.
8. Serve hot and enjoy!

Tip:

- Add visual appeal by using a variety of bell pepper hues.
  Feel free to add other ingredients to the filling, such as chopped spinach, sun-dried tomatoes, or pine nuts.
- For a vegan version, leave off the Parmesan cheese or replace it with nutritional yeast.
- Refrigerate the leftover filled mushrooms and reheat them in the oven or microwave.

Health Benefits for Fatty Liver:

- Quinoa is an excellent source of plant-based protein, including all nine necessary amino acids. It is also high in fiber, which may help with digestion and blood sugar regulation, both of which are critical in fatty liver management.
- Mushrooms are low in calories yet abundant in antioxidants, vitamins, and minerals. They may have anti-inflammatory qualities that benefit liver function. Olive oil, when taken in moderation, is a healthy fat rich in monounsaturated fatty acids, which may help prevent liver fat formation and inflammation.
- This dish is minimal in saturated fat and has no additional sweets, making it a healthy alternative for those with fatty liver disease. However, portion management is still critical, especially when managing calorie intake.

Edamame Salad

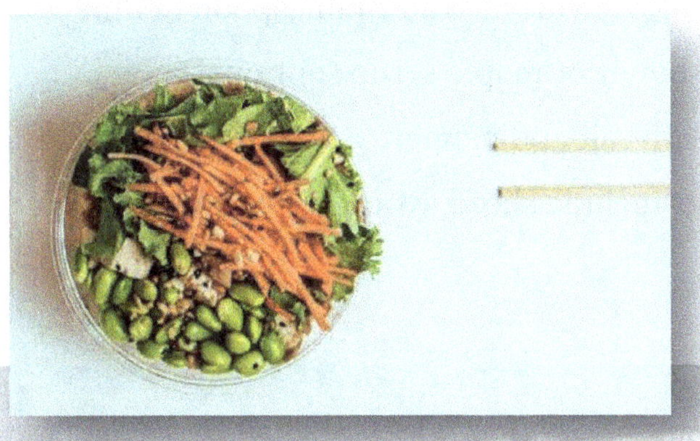

Prep Time: 10 minutes

Cooking Time: 5 minutes (to blanch edamame)

Total time: 15 minutes

Serving size: 4

Nutritional Data (Per Serving)

- Calories: 180 kcal.
- 12 grams of protein.
- Fat: 8g
- Carbohydrate: 16g
- Fiber: 6 grams.
- Sugar: 3 grams.
- Sodium: 200 mg.

Ingredients:

- 2 cups shelled edamame (frozen or fresh) and 1 cup halved cherry tomatoes.

- Combine 1/2 cup diced cucumber, 1/4 cup chopped red onion, 1/4 cup chopped fresh cilantro or parsley, and 2 tablespoons extra virgin olive oil.
- Use 2 teaspoons of rice vinegar and 1 tablespoon of lime juice.
- One teaspoon of honey or maple syrup (optional)
- Season to taste with salt and pepper.
- Optional toppings include sliced avocado, sesame seeds, and crumbled feta cheese.

Directions:

1. Heat a saucepan of water to a boil. Add the shelled edamame and blanch for 3–4 minutes. To halt the cooking process, drain and rinse well with cold water. Drain well.
2. In a large mixing bowl, add blanched edamame, cherry tomatoes, cucumber, red onion, and chopped cilantro or parsley.
3. In a small mixing bowl, combine the extra virgin olive oil, rice vinegar, lime juice, honey or maple syrup (if using), salt, and pepper to prepare the dressing.
4. Pour the dressing over the salad ingredients and mix until equally distributed.
5. Taste and adjust seasoning as required.
6. Before serving, garnish the salad with sliced avocado, sesame seeds, or crumbled feta cheese.
7. Serve immediately, or chill until ready to serve.

Tip:

- Thaw frozen edamame before blanching.
  To enhance the taste, add diced bell pepper, shredded carrots, or chopped scallions to the salad.
- This salad may be prepared ahead of time and kept in the fridge for up to two days. However, to avoid browning, add the avocado right before serving.
  For a distinct taste profile, season the dressing with chili flakes or soy sauce.

Health Benefits for Fatty Liver:

- Edamame is high in plant protein and includes necessary amino acids. It is also high in fiber, which may help anage blood sugar and promote digestion, both of which are crucial in the treatment of fatty liver disease.
- This salad's veggies, including cherry tomatoes, cucumber, and red onion, are low in calories and high in vitamins, minerals, and antioxidants, all of which may help decrease inflammation and promote liver function.
- The olive oil used in the dressing is a healthy fat rich in monounsaturated fatty acids, which may help to prevent liver fat formation and inflammation. Incorporating salads like this one into your diet may aid in weight control and liver health by providing nutrient-dense, low-calorie alternatives.

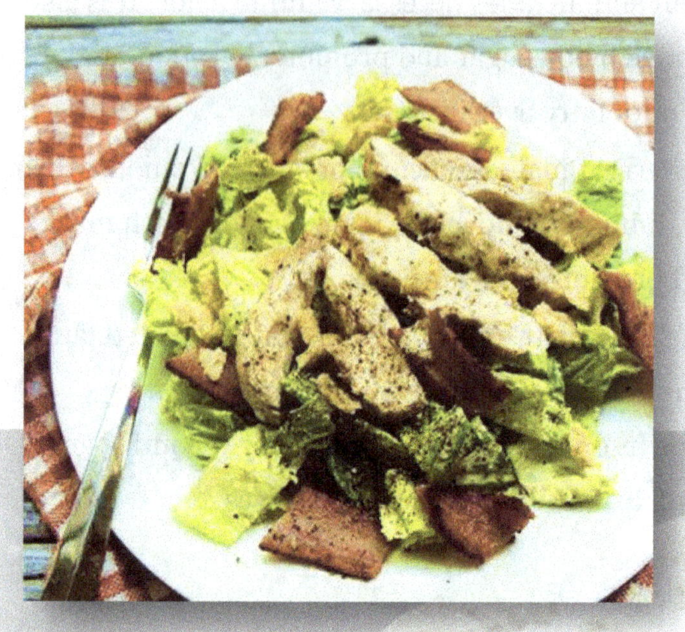

CHAPTER 3

SOUPS AND SALADS

Soups and salads can play a crucial role in managing fatty liver disease due to their nutritious ingredients and potential health benefits. For soups, opting for broth-based varieties with plenty of vegetables and lean proteins can provide essential nutrients while keeping fat content low. Incorporating salads rich in leafy greens, colorful vegetables, lean proteins, and healthy fats like avocado or olive oil can support liver health by promoting weight management and providing essential vitamins, minerals, and antioxidants. Choosing recipes low in added sugars, refined carbohydrates, and unhealthy fats can further aid in managing fatty liver disease. However, it's essential to consider individual dietary needs and consult with a healthcare professional for personalized dietary recommendations.

Lentil Soup

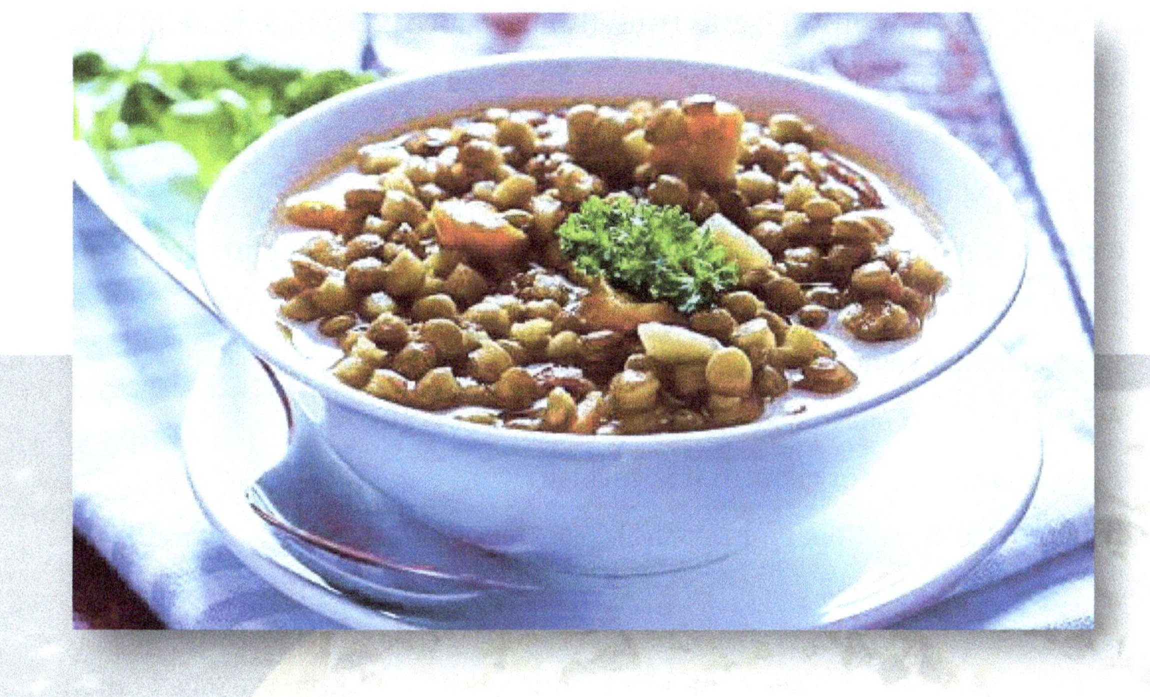

Prep Time: 10 minutes

Cooking Time: 40 minutes.

Total time: 50 minutes

Serving size: 6

Nutritional Data (Per Serving):

- Calories: 250 kcal.
- 15 grams of protein.
- Fat: 2g
- Carbohydrate: 45 grams
- Fiber: 15g; sugar: 5g.
- Sodium: 500 mg.

Ingredients:

- 1 cup dry green or brown lentils (rinsed and drained), 1 chopped onion, 2 diced carrots, and 2 diced celery stalks.
- 3 garlic cloves minced
- One can (14 ounces) of chopped tomatoes
- 6 cups vegetable or chicken broth, 1 teaspoon ground cumin, and 1 teaspoon ground coriander.
- 1/2 teaspoon of smoked paprika.
- Add salt and pepper to taste. Use 2 tablespoons of olive oil.
- Freshly cut parsley or cilantro (for garnish)
- Lemon wedges (optional for serving).

Directions:

1. Warm the olive oil in a big saucepan over medium heat. Combine the diced onion, carrots, and celery. Cook for about 5-7 minutes, or until the veggies have softened.
2. Combine the minced garlic, cumin, coriander, and smoked paprika. Cook for another 1-2 minutes, until fragrant.
3. Stir in the rinsed lentils, chopped tomatoes (with liquids), and stock. Heat the soup to a boil.
4. Reduce the heat to low, cover, and let simmer for approximately 30 minutes, or until the lentils are cooked.
5. Season the soup with salt and pepper as desired.
6. For a smoother texture, combine a part of the soup with an immersion blender or transfer it to a blender and puree before returning it to the pot.
7. Serve hot and garnish with fresh parsley or cilantro. Serve with lemon wedges for an added blast of citrus flavor.

Tips:

- Lentils provide plant-based protein and fiber, making this soup a healthy alternative for those with fatty liver disease. Fiber regulates blood sugar levels and assists digestion, both of which are critical for treating fatty liver.
- To reduce the salt content, use low-sodium broth or make your own broth at home.
- Feel free to add more veggies to the soup, such as bell peppers, spinach, or kale.
- Leftover soup may be refrigerated for up to four days or frozen for longer storage.
- Reheat gently on the stove or in the microwave before serving.

Health Benefits for Fatty Liver:

- Lentils are high in fiber, which helps manage blood sugar and digestion. This may be advantageous for those with fatty liver disease since it helps control insulin resistance and lowers the risk of future liver damage.
- Vegetables such as carrots, celery, and tomatoes are high in vitamins, minerals, and antioxidants, which promote overall liver function and may help decrease inflammation caused by fatty liver disease.
- Using olive oil instead of saturated fats such as butter or lard may help decrease cholesterol and minimize liver fat formation, resulting in better liver function.
- This lentil soup dish is low in saturated fat and has no additional sweeteners, making it a healthy choice for those with fatty liver disease. However, portion management is still critical, especially when managing calorie intake.

Kale and White Bean Soup

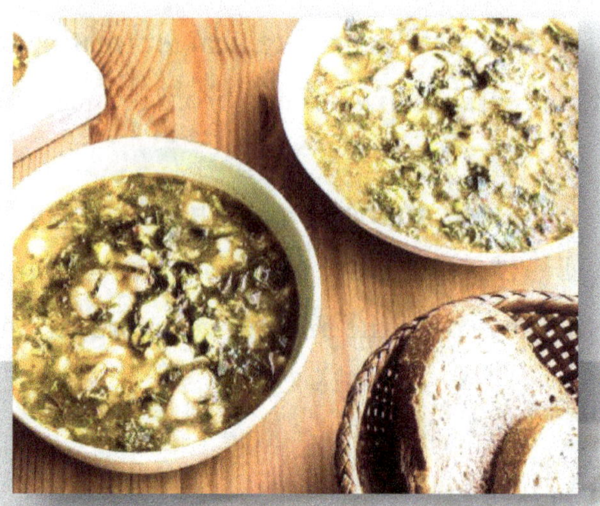

Prep Time: 15 minutes

Cooking Time: 30 minutes.

Total time: 45 minutes

Servings: 4

Nutritional Data (Per Serving):

- Calories: 250 kcal.
- 12 grams of protein.
- Fat: 6g
- Carbohydrate: 40 grams
- Fiber: 10g; sugar: 4g.
- Sodium: 600 mg.

Ingredients:

- To prepare, combine 1 tablespoon olive oil, 1 diced onion, and 2 minced garlic cloves.

- Dice two carrots and two celery stalks.
- 4 cups vegetable or chicken broth and 2 cups water.
- 2 cans (15 oz) of white beans (such as cannellini or Great Northern), drained and rinsed
- 1 bunch chopped kale, 1 teaspoon dried thyme, salt and pepper to taste, and optional red pepper flakes for spiciness.
  grated Parmesan cheese (optional garnish)

Directions:

1. Warm the olive oil in a big saucepan over medium heat. Combine the diced onion, garlic, carrots, and celery. Cook for about 5-7 minutes, or until the veggies have softened.

2. Combine the vegetable or chicken broth, water, white beans, chopped kale, and dried thyme in the saucepan. Heat the soup to a boil.

3. Reduce the heat to low, cover, and cook for 20–25 minutes, or until the veggies are cooked and the kale has wilted.

4. To taste, season the soup with salt, pepper, and red pepper flakes (if using).

5. Serve hot, topped with grated Parmesan cheese if preferred.

Tips:

- Kale is a nutrient-dense leafy green vegetable high in vitamins, minerals, and antioxidants, making it an excellent addition to any liver-healthy diet. Its high fiber content may aid in digestion and blood sugar regulation, both of which are critical in the treatment of fatty liver disease.
- White beans are high in plant-based protein and fiber, which may help people with fatty liver disease improve satiety and weight control.
- To limit salt intake, use low-sodium broth or create your own broth at home.
- This soup is readily customizable by adding other veggies, such as chopped tomatoes, spinach, or zucchini.
- Leftover soup may be refrigerated for up to four days or frozen for longer storage. Reheat gently on the stove or in the microwave before serving.

Health Benefits for Fatty Liver:

- This soup's nutrient-dense blend of kale and white beans promotes liver wellness. Both kale and white beans include fiber, vitamins, minerals, and antioxidants, which may help decrease inflammation and improve liver function.
- The olive oil used in the soup contains beneficial monounsaturated fats, which may help to prevent liver fat buildup and inflammation associated with fatty liver disease.
- A plant-based diet high in kale and white beans may help with weight control and insulin sensitivity, both of which are helpful in treating fatty liver disease.

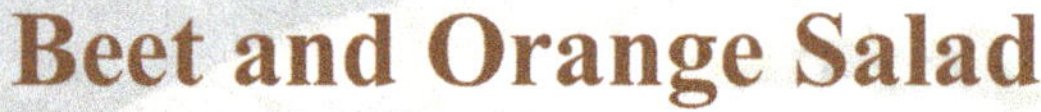

Beet and Orange Salad

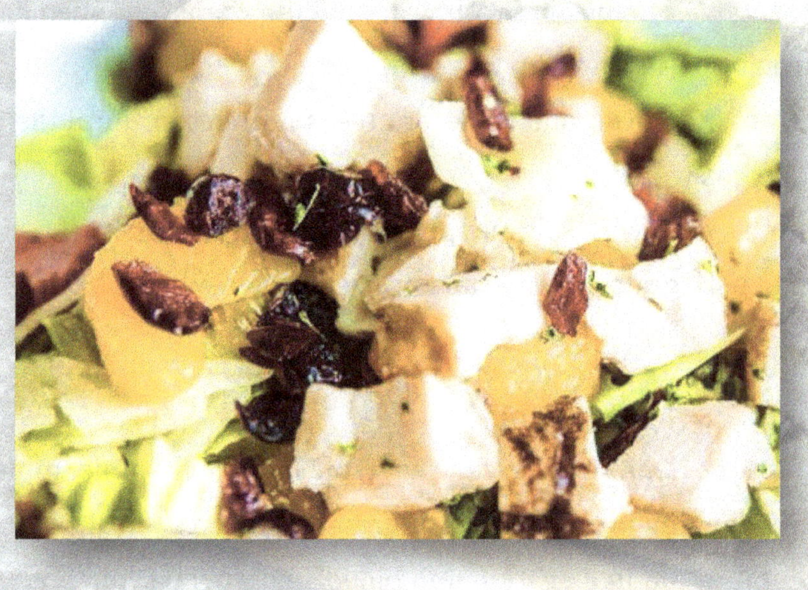

Prep Time: 15 minutes

Cooking Time: 45 minutes (for beet roasting)

Total time: 60 minutes

Serving size: 4

Nutritional Data (Per Serving):

- Calories: 150 kcal.
- 3 grams of protein.
- Fat: 2g
- Carbohydrate: 32 grams
- Fiber: 6 grams.
- Sugar: 22 grams.
- Sodium: 200 mg.

Ingredients:

- Four medium beets, roasted, peeled, and sliced
- Two oranges, peeled and sliced
- 1/4 cup chopped walnuts or pecans (optional).
- Two cups of baby spinach or mixed greens
- 1/4 cup crumbled goat or feta cheese (optional).
- 2 tablespoons extra virgin olive oil, 1 tablespoon balsamic vinegar, and 1 teaspoon honey or maple syrup.
- Season to taste with salt and pepper.
- Garnish with fresh parsley or mint leaves.

Directions:

1. If not previously roasted, preheat the oven to 400°F (200°C). Wrap each beet separately in aluminum foil and lay it on a baking pan. Roast for approximately 45 minutes, or until fork-tender. Allow the beets to cool before peeling and slicing them into rounds.

2. In a small mixing bowl, combine the extra virgin olive oil, balsamic vinegar, honey or maple syrup, salt, and pepper to prepare the dressing.

3. Place the baby spinach or mixed greens on a serving dish or individual plates.

4. Garnish the greens with roasted beet and orange slices.

5. Drizzle the dressing over the salad.

6. If using, top the salad with chopped walnuts or pecans, as well as crumbled feta or goat cheese.

7. Garnish with fresh parsley or mint leaves.

8. Serve immediately and enjoy!

Tip:

- To save time, use pre-cooked or canned beets. Just remember to drain and rinse canned beets before using them.
- If you like a nuttier taste, toast the chopped walnuts or pecans in a dry pan over medium heat for a few minutes until fragrant before mixing them into the salad.
- For a vegan version, leave off the cheese or use a dairy-free replacement.
- Leftover salad may be refrigerated for up to two days. To avoid soggy greens, keep the dressing separate until ready to serve.

Health Benefits for Fatty Liver:

- Beets are high in antioxidants, notably betalains, which have anti-inflammatory qualities and may help decrease liver inflammation caused by fatty liver disease.
- Oranges include vitamin C, which is important for liver health because it promotes the development of glutathione, a potent antioxidant that aids in liver detoxification.
- Spinach and other leafy greens are rich in fiber and low in calories, making them excellent for weight control, which is especially important for those with fatty liver disease.
- Nuts such as walnuts and pecans provide good fats and protein, which may improve satiety and minimize overeating, aiding weight control attempts.
- However, because of the high calorie content, portion management is essential.
- A salad with colorful fruits, vegetables, nuts, and seeds has a range of nutrients that promote overall liver function and may help minimize the risk of liver disease development.

Quinoa and Black Bean Salad

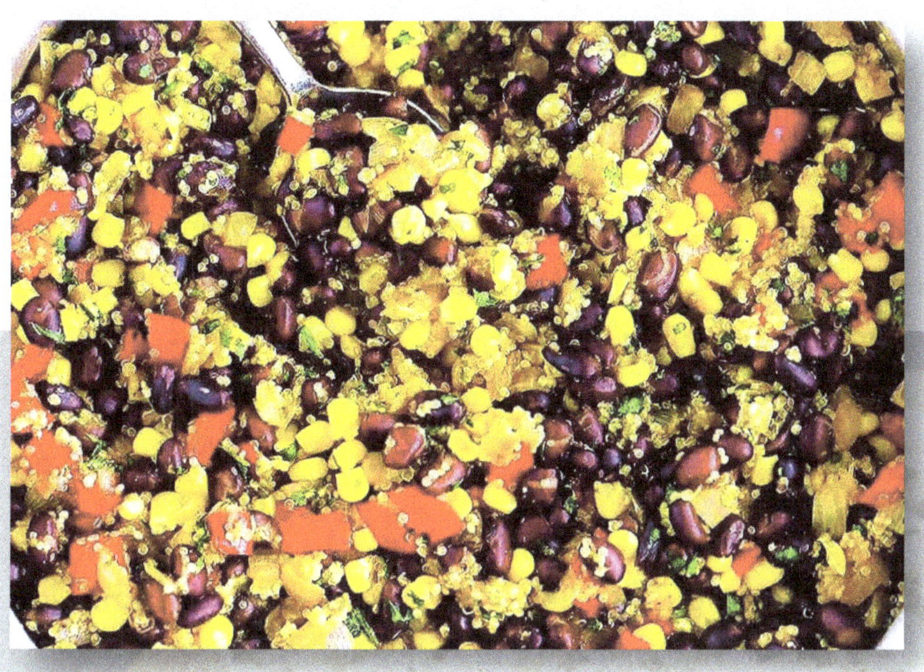

Prep Time: 15 minutes

Cooking Time: 15 minutes.

Total Time: 30 minutes

Servings: 4

Nutritional Data (Per Serving):

- Calories: 300 kcal.
- 12 grams of protein.
- Fat: 10g
- Carbohydrate: 40 grams
- Fiber: 10g; sugar: 2g.
- Sodium: 400 mg.

Ingredients:

- To prepare, combine 1 cup washed quinoa, 2 cups water or vegetable broth, and 1 can (15 oz) drained and rinsed black beans.
- One red bell pepper, chopped
- Half cup corn kernels (fresh, canned, or frozen)
- 1/4 cup diced red onion, 1/4 cup chopped fresh cilantro, and 1 diced avocado.
- To prepare, combine 1 lime juice, 2 tablespoons extra virgin olive oil, 1 teaspoon ground cumin, salt, and pepper to taste.
- Optional toppings include diced tomatoes, sliced jalapeños, and crumbled feta cheese.

Directions:

1. In a medium saucepan, mix the quinoa, water, or vegetable broth. Bring to a boil, then lower to a low heat, cover, and simmer for 12–15 minutes, or until the quinoa is cooked and the liquid has been absorbed. Remove from heat and let cool.

2. In a large mixing bowl, mix together the cooked quinoa, black beans, diced bell pepper, corn kernels, diced red onion, and cilantro.

3. In a small mixing bowl, combine the lime juice, extra virgin olive oil, ground cumin, salt, and pepper to prepare the dressing.

4. Pour the dressing over the quinoa-black bean combination. Toss everything until it is well covered.

5. Gently fold in the cubed avocado.

6. Taste and adjust seasoning as needed.

7. Serve chilled or at room temperature. Optional toppings include chopped tomatoes, sliced jalapeños, or crumbled feta cheese.

Tip:

- You may modify this salad by adding veggies such as diced tomatoes, shredded carrots, or chopped spinach.
- For added taste, add a dab of spicy sauce or chili powder to the dressing.

- Leftover quinoa and black bean salad may be refrigerated in an airtight container for up to three days. The avocado may color somewhat over time, but it is still safe to consume.
- This salad may be served as the main course for a light lunch or supper, or as a side dish with grilled meats or seafood.

Health Benefits:

- Quinoa is a nutrient-rich whole grain with high protein and fiber content, providing a healthy and fulfilling basis for this salad. Fiber improves digestion and may help manage blood sugar levels, which is essential for treating fatty liver disease.
- Black beans are rich in plant-based protein, fiber, and antioxidants. They may help decrease cholesterol and enhance heart health, which is good for those who have fatty liver disease.
- Avocado contains beneficial monounsaturated fats, which may help prevent liver fat buildup and inflammation caused by fatty liver disease. Avocados are also high in vitamins, minerals, and antioxidants, which promote general liver function.
- The bright veggies in this salad, including bell pepper, maize, and red onion, provide critical vitamins, minerals, and antioxidants that may help decrease inflammation and enhance liver function.

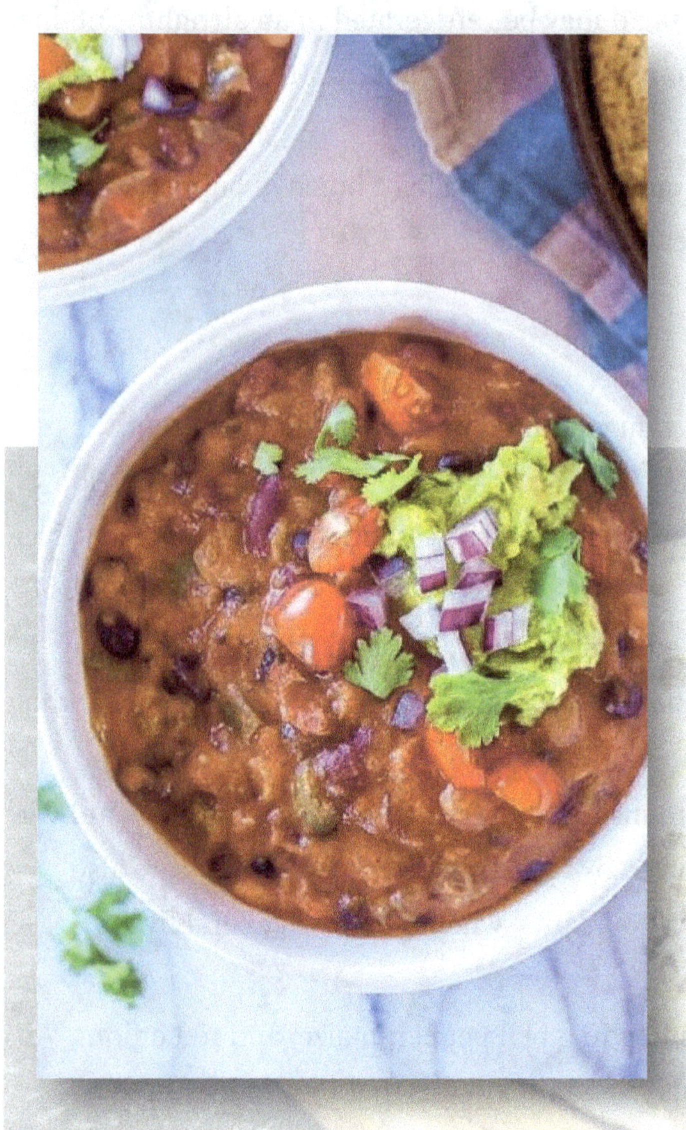

CHAPTER 4

MAIN COURSES

Main courses for those with fatty liver disease should include lean protein sources, lots of veggies, whole grains, and healthy fats. Here is a little introduction:

The main courses designed for fatty liver health focus on nutrient-dense items that promote liver function and general well-being. Grilled chicken, fish, tofu, and lentils are all lean protein sources that supply important amino acids without adding too much saturated fat. Incorporating a range of colorful veggies into major meals not only adds taste and texture, but it also provides antioxidants and fiber, which help with digestion and inflammation. Whole grains such as quinoa, brown rice, and whole wheat pasta include complex carbs that give long-lasting energy and help manage blood sugar levels. Healthy fats from sources such as olive oil, avocado, and almonds promote heart health and may help prevent liver fat formation. Individuals suffering from fatty liver disease may improve their liver health while eating tasty and gratifying meals by choosing balanced and healthy main dishes.

Baked salmon with lemon and dill

Prep Time: 10 minutes

Cooking Time: 15 minutes.

Total time: 25 minutes

Serving size: 4

Nutritional Data (Per Serving):

- Calories: 250 kcal.
- Protein: 30 grams.
- Fat: 12g
- Carbohydrate: 2g
- Fiber: 0 grams
- Sugar: 0 grams
- Sodium: 300 mg.

Ingredients:

- 4 salmon fillets (about 6 ounces each), skin-on or skinless.
  Ingredients: 2 tablespoons olive oil, 2 teaspoons fresh lemon juice.
- 2 garlic cloves, minced
- 2 tablespoons chopped fresh dill;
- season to taste with salt and pepper;
- Garnish with lemon slices and fresh dill.

Directions:

1. Preheat the oven to 400°F (200°C). Line a baking sheet with parchment paper or gently coat it with olive oil.

2. In a small bowl, combine the olive oil, lemon juice, minced garlic, fresh dill, salt, and pepper.

3. Arrange the salmon fillets on the prepared baking sheet, skin side down, if applicable.

4. Distribute the lemon and dill mixture evenly over the salmon fillets, ensuring they are fully covered.

5. Marinate the salmon for approximately 10 minutes at room temperature to enable the flavors to combine.

6. Bake the salmon in the preheated oven for 12–15 minutes, or until it is well cooked and readily flaked with a fork. The salmon's internal temperature should reach 145°F (63°C).

7. After baking, take the salmon from the oven and allow it to rest for a few minutes.

8. Serve the baked salmon hot, topped with lemon slices and more fresh dill, if preferred.

Tip:

- Select firm, vivid pink salmon fillets for optimal results. If using frozen salmon, let it defrost in the fridge overnight before cooking.
- Feel free to alter the seasoning to your liking. You may adjust the amount of garlic, lemon juice, and dill to your preference.
- To keep the salmon from drying out when baking, don't overcook. To check for doneness, carefully put a fork into the thickest section of the fillet. It should flake quickly and be opaque.
- For a full and balanced dinner, pair the baked salmon with your favorite side dishes, such as roasted vegetables, steaming rice, or a crisp salad.

Health Benefits for Fatty Liver:

- Salmon is high in omega-3 fatty acids, which have anti-inflammatory qualities that may help people with fatty liver disease by lowering inflammation and improving liver function.
- In this dish, the garlic contains chemicals that may help protect the liver from injury and aid in detoxification.

- Dill contains antioxidants and vitamins, including vitamin C and vitamin A, which may help promote liver function and prevent oxidative stress.
- In general, this Baked Salmon with Lemon and Dill dish is a healthy and tasty alternative for those with fatty liver disease, including a variety of essential nutrients and tastes that may help with liver function and general well-being.

Turkey Meatloaf with Mushroom

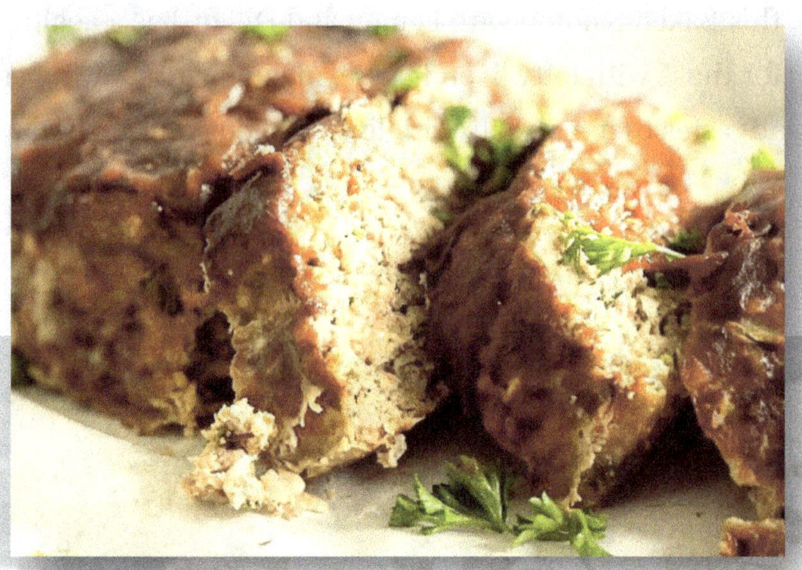

Prep Time: 15 min.

Cooking Time: 1 hour

Total time: 1 hour, 15 minutes

Servings: 6

Nutritional Data (Per Serving, Including Gravy):

- Calories: 300 kcal.
- Protein: 25 grams.
- Fat: 15g
- Carbohydrate: 15 grams
- Fiber: 3 grams.
- Sugar: 5 grams.
- Sodium: 600 mg.

Ingredients for Turkey Meatloaf:

- 1 pound of ground turkey, ideally lean.
- 1/2 cup breadcrumbs, whole wheat or gluten-free.
- 1/4 cup grated Parmesan cheese, 1/4 cup milk (or unsweetened almond milk).
- Add 1/4 cup chopped onion and 1/4 cup chopped bell pepper.
- 2 garlic cloves minced
- One tablespoon of Worcestershire sauce.
- 1 teaspoon dried thyme; 1 teaspoon dried oregano.
- Season to taste with salt and pepper.
- Grease with a cooking spray or olive oil.

Ingredients for Mushroom Gravy:

- 8 oz. of mushrooms (cremini or button), sliced
- Two tablespoons of butter or olive oil
- Two tablespoons of all-purpose flour (or gluten-free flour)
- Use 1 cup low-sodium chicken or veggie broth and 1/4 cup milk (or unsweetened almond milk).
- Add salt and pepper to taste.

Directions:

1. Preheat the oven to 375°F (190°C). Coat a loaf pan with cooking spray or olive oil.

2. In a large mixing bowl, mix together the ground turkey, breadcrumbs, grated Parmesan cheese, milk, diced onion, chopped bell pepper, minced garlic, Worcestershire sauce, dried thyme, dried oregano, salt, and pepper. Mix until well mixed.

3. Pour the turkey mixture into a prepared loaf pan and form it into a loaf shape.

4. Cook the turkey meatloaf in a preheated oven for 45–50 minutes, or until the internal temperature reaches 165°F (74°C) and the top becomes golden brown.

5. While the meatloaf bakes, make the mushroom gravy. In a pan, melt the butter or olive oil over medium heat. Cook the sliced mushrooms until soft and caramelized, approximately 5-7 minutes.

6. Sprinkle the flour over the mushrooms and toss to evenly coat. Cook for another 1–2 minutes.

7. Slowly add the chicken or vegetable broth, stirring frequently to avoid lumps from forming.

8. Add the milk and boil for another 5 minutes, or until the gravy thickens. Season with salt and pepper, to taste.

9. After the turkey meatloaf has finished baking, let it rest for a few minutes before slicing.

10. Serve the sliced turkey meatloaf with mushroom gravy on top.

Tips:

- Use ground turkey with a low fat level (approximately 93% lean) to make the meatloaf moist without adding too much fat.
- For added taste and nutrition, try adding grated carrots or zucchini to the meatloaf recipe.
- To make a gluten-free meatloaf and gravy, use gluten-free breadcrumbs and flour.
- Leftover turkey meatloaf may be refrigerated in an airtight container for up to three days. Heat gently in the oven or microwave before serving.
- For a full and fulfilling supper, pair the meatloaf with your favorite side dishes, such as mashed potatoes, roasted vegetables, or a green salad.

Health Benefits:

- Turkey is a lean protein source with lower saturated fat than beef, making it a better choice for those with fatty liver disease.
- Mushrooms are low in calories and high in antioxidants, vitamins, and minerals, including vitamin D and selenium, which may help with liver health and inflammation.

- Using whole wheat breadcrumbs and veggies in the meatloaf increases the dish's fiber content, which promotes digestion and regulates blood sugar levels.
- The homemade mushroom gravy provides taste without adding too much fat and may be prepared using low-sodium broth to minimize salt consumption, which is good for those who have fatty liver disease.

Lemon Herb Chicken with Roasted Vegetables

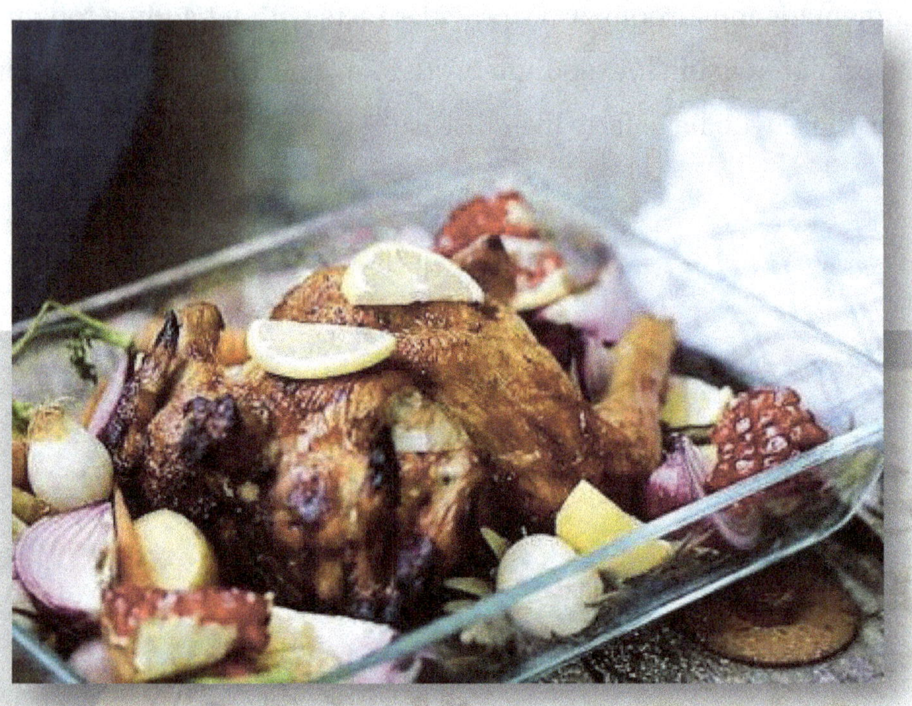

Preparation time: 15 minutes

Cooking time: 25 minutes

Total time: 40 minutes

Serving size: 4

Nutritional Data (Per Serving):

- Calories: 300 kcal.
- 25 grams of protein.
- Fat: 10g
- Carbohydrate: 20 grams
- Fiber: 5g, sugar: 8g.
- Sodium: 400 mg.

Ingredients for Lemon Herb Chicken:

- Four boneless and skinless chicken breasts
- 2 tablespoons olive oil, 2 teaspoons fresh lemon juice.
- 2 garlic cloves, minced
- Use 1 teaspoon dried thyme and 1 teaspoon dry rosemary.
- Add salt and pepper to taste.
- Garnish with lemon slices.

Ingredients for Roasted Vegetables:

- 2 cups mixed veggies (such as bell peppers, zucchini, cherry tomatoes, and red onion), chopped
- One tablespoon of olive oil.
- 1 teaspoon dry Italian seasoning (or a mixture of dried basil, oregano, and thyme)
- Add salt and pepper to taste.

Directions:

1. Preheat the oven to 400°F (200°C). Line a baking sheet with parchment or aluminum foil.

2. In a small mixing bowl, combine the olive oil, fresh lemon juice, minced garlic, dried thyme, dried rosemary, salt, and pepper to make the marinade for the chicken.

3. Transfer the chicken breasts to a shallow plate or resalable plastic bag. Pour the marinade over the chicken and make sure it's uniformly covered. Allow the chicken to marinade for at least 15 minutes or up to an hour in the refrigerator.

4. While the chicken marinates, prepare the veggies. Toss the chopped veggies in a large mixing basin with olive oil, dry Italian seasoning, salt, and pepper until well covered.

5. Arrange the seasoned veggies in a single layer on the prepared baking sheet.

6. Remove the chicken breasts from the marinade and put them on a baking sheet with the veggies.

7. Bake in the preheated oven for 20–25 minutes, or until the chicken is done and the veggies are soft and faintly caramelized.

8. After cooking, remove the baking sheet from the oven and allow the chicken to rest for a few minutes before slicing.

9. For a blast of freshness, serve the lemon herb chicken with the roasted veggies, topped with lemon slices.

Tip:

- Choose uniformly thick chicken breasts for even cooking.
- Feel free to vary the veggies depending on your tastes and what is in season. You may also include other veggies like broccoli, carrots, or asparagus.
- To avoid drying out the chicken, don't overcook it. Use a meat thermometer to verify the chicken's internal temperature is 165°F (74°C).
- Leftover lemon herb chicken and roasted veggies may be refrigerated in separate airtight containers for up to three days. Heat gently in the oven or microwave before serving.

Health benefits:

- Chicken is a lean source of protein that has less saturated fat than red meat, making it a heart-healthy choice for those with fatty liver disease.
- Lemon juice boosts the dish's vitamin C content, which aids in immunological function and iron absorption from plant-based diets.
- Garlic and herbs such as thyme and rosemary not only improve the taste of the chicken, but they also contain antioxidants and anti-inflammatory characteristics that benefit liver health.
- Roasted veggies are high in fiber, vitamins, and minerals, which are necessary components for digestion and general health. The combination of colorful vegetables contains a range of antioxidants, which help protect cells from harm and decrease inflammation in the body, especially in the liver.

Vegan Chili

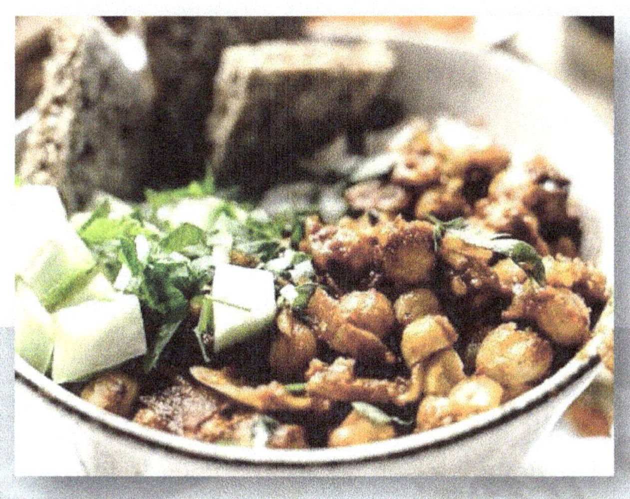

Prep Time: 15 minutes

Cooking Time: 30 minutes

Total Time: 45 minutes

Serving Size: 6

Nutritional Data (Per Serving):

- Calories: 250 kcal.
- 12 grams of protein.
- Fat: 5g
- Carbohydrate: 40 grams
- Fiber: 12g; sugar: 8g.
- Sodium: 600 mg.

Ingredients:

- One tablespoon of olive oil.

- 1 onion, diced

- 2 garlic cloves, minced

- One chopped bell pepper.

- Dice one zucchini and one carrot.

- One can (15 oz) of kidney beans, drained and rinsed

- one can (15 oz) of black beans, drained and rinsed

- One (15-ounce) can of chopped tomatoes

- Add 1 cup of vegetable broth and 2 teaspoons of chili powder.

- Add 1 teaspoon cumin and 1 teaspoon paprika.

- Season to taste with salt and pepper.

- Optional toppings include chopped cilantro, avocado slices, shredded cheese, and sour cream.

Directions:

1. In a large saucepan, heat the olive oil over medium heat. Sauté the diced onion and garlic until softened, approximately 5 minutes.

2. Add the chopped bell pepper, zucchini, and carrot to the saucepan. Cook for a further 5 minutes, until the veggies are somewhat tender.

3. Add the drained and rinsed kidney beans, black beans, chopped tomatoes, vegetable broth, chili powder, cumin, paprika, salt, and pepper to the saucepan. Stir to mix.

4. Bring the chili to a boil, then decrease the heat to low and stew uncovered for 20–25 minutes, stirring regularly.

5. Once the chili has thickened and the flavors have merged, taste and adjust seasoning as needed.

6. Serve the vegetarian chili hot, topped with chopped cilantro, avocado slices, shredded cheese, or a dollop of sour cream, as preferred.

Tip:

- Customize the chili by adding veggies or changing the amount of spiciness using chili powder.

- Textured vegetable protein (TVP), lentils, or quinoa may be added to the chili to boost the protein content.
- Leftover vegetarian chili may be refrigerated for up to four days or frozen for extended storage. Reheat gently on the stove or in the microwave before serving.

Health Benefits:

- Vegetarian chili has high fiber, which promotes digestion and regulates blood sugar levels, making it excellent for those with fatty liver disease.
- Beans are high in plant-based protein and soluble fiber, which help decrease cholesterol and improve heart health.
- The diversity of vegetables in the chili contains necessary vitamins, minerals, and antioxidants that promote liver health and decrease inflammation in the body.

Stir-fried tofu with broccoli and brown rice

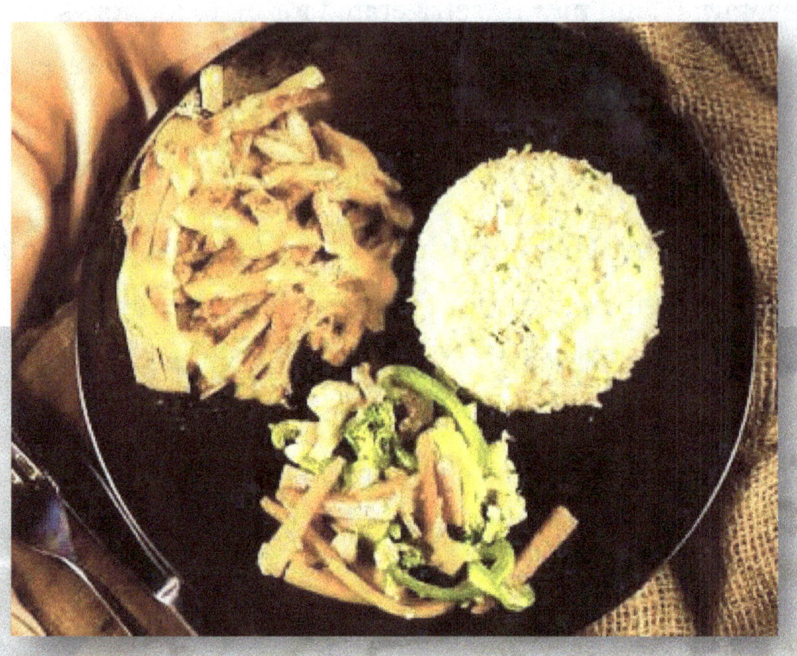

Prep Time: 15 minutes

Cooking Time: 15 minutes

Total Time: 30 minutes Serving Size: 4

Nutritional Data (Per Serving):

- Calories: 300 kcal.
- 15 grams of protein.
- Fat: 10g
- Carbohydrate: 40 grams
- Fiber: 6g, sugar: 4g.
- Sodium: 400 mg.

Ingredients:

- 1 block (14 oz) of firm tofu, pressed and cubed 2 tablespoons soy sauce (or tamari for gluten-free)
- 1 tablespoon sesame oil and 2 minced garlic cloves.
- 1 tablespoon grated ginger, 1 head broccoli chopped into florets.
- 1 bell pepper, chopped
- Prepare 1 julienned carrot, 2 sliced green onions, and cooked brown rice for serving.
- Optional garnishes include sesame seeds and chopped cilantro.

Directions:

1. In a large skillet or wok, heat the sesame oil over medium heat. Sauté minced garlic and grated ginger for 1-2 minutes, until aromatic.

2. Add the cubed tofu to the pan and stir-fry for 5-7 minutes, or until browned on both sides.

3. Add the soy sauce and simmer for a further 2-3 minutes, enabling the tofu to absorb the flavors.

4. Place the broccoli florets, sliced bell pepper, and julienned carrot in the pan. Stir-fry the veggies for 3–4 minutes, until they are soft yet still crisp.

5. Once the veggies have cooked to your taste, remove the pan from the heat.

6. Serve the stir-fried tofu and veggies hot with prepared brown rice.

7. Optional garnishes include chopped green onions, sesame seeds, and cilantro.

Tip:

- Pressing tofu before cooking removes unnecessary moisture and enhances flavor absorption.
- For extra flavor and nutrients, mix in other veggies such as snow peas, mushrooms, or bok choy.
- To add a spicy touch to the stir-fry sauce, mix with chili flakes or sriracha.
- Leftover stir-fried tofu and veggies may be refrigerated for up to three days.
- Reheat gently in a pan or microwave before serving.

Health benefits:

- Tofu is a plant-based protein with minimal saturated fat and cholesterol, making it a healthier alternative to animal protein sources.
- Broccoli is high in antioxidants and includes chemicals that aid in liver detoxification, making it useful for those with fatty liver disease.
- Brown rice is a complete grain rich in fiber and complex carbs, which provide long-lasting energy and aid digestion. It also includes B vitamins and minerals like selenium and magnesium, which promote general health and well-being.

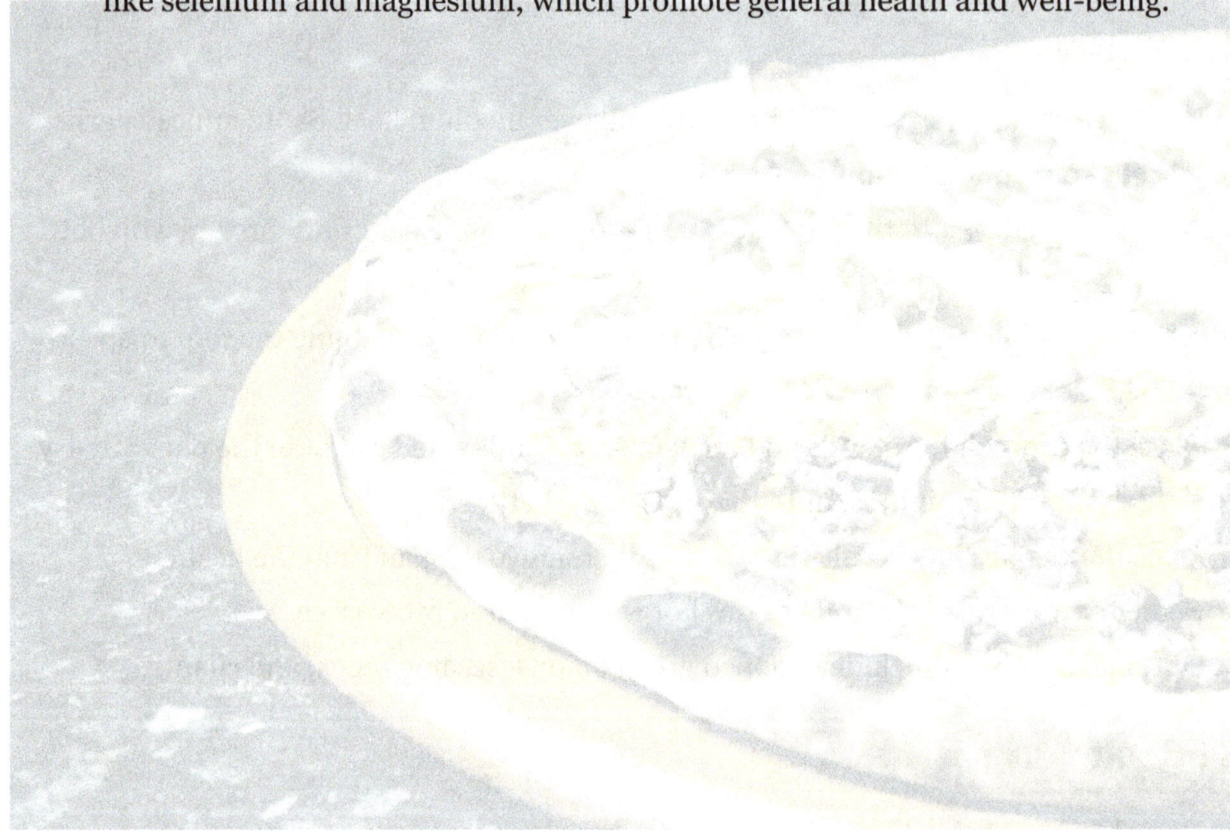

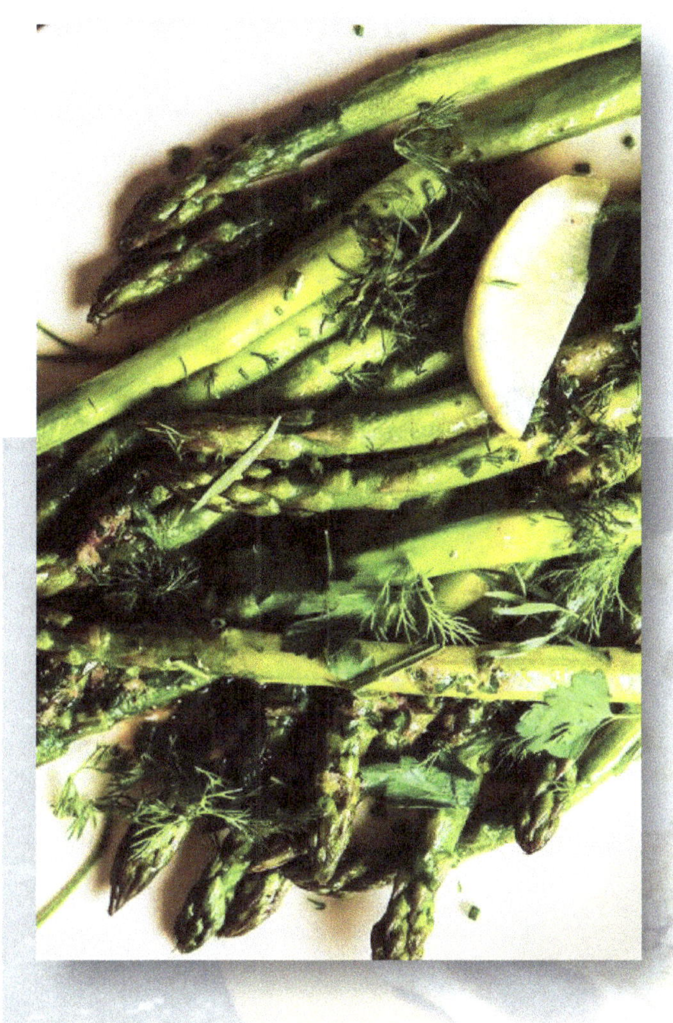

<h1 style="text-align:center">CHAPTER 5</h1>

<h1 style="text-align:center">SIDE DISHES</h1>

Side dishes and accompaniments are crucial components of a well-balanced dinner, particularly for those who have fatty livers. These additions not only improve the tastes and textures of a meal but also provide a chance to include nutrient-dense foods that promote liver function. Choosing sides and accompaniments low in saturated fats, salt, and added sweets will help you manage fatty liver disease successfully. Think of colorful veggies, whole grains, legumes, and healthy fats like avocado and olive oil. By concentrating on nutrient-dense selections and exercising portion control, you can create meals that improve liver health and overall well-being.

Garlic-roasted Brussels sprouts

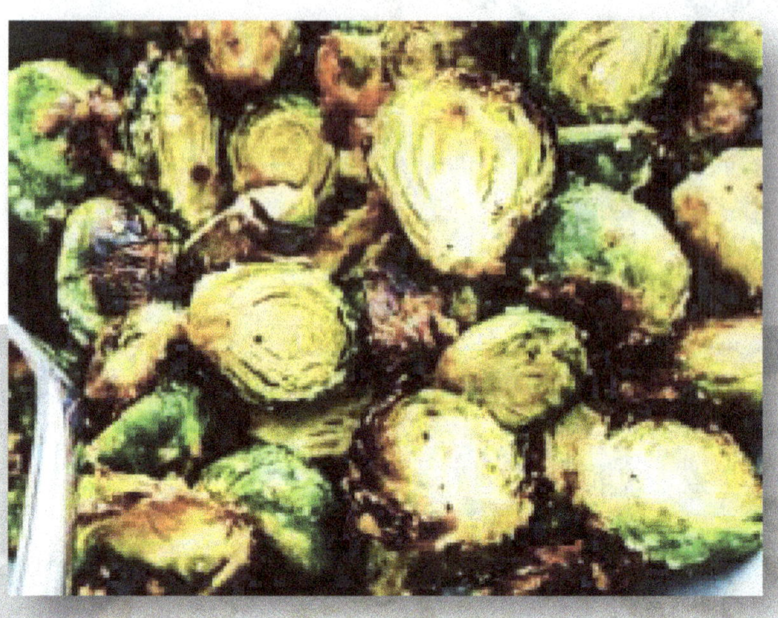

Prep Time: 10 minutes

Cooking Time: 25 minutes.

Total time: 35 minutes

Serving size: 4

Nutritional Data (Per Serving):

- Calories: 100 kcal.
- 4 grams of protein
- Fat: 5g
- carbs: 12g
- Fiber: 4 grams.
- Sugar: 2 grams.
- Sodium: 200 mg.

Ingredients:

- 1 lb. trimmed and halved Brussels sprouts, 2 tablespoons olive oil, and 3 chopped garlic cloves.
- 1 teaspoon dried thyme (or 1 tablespoon of fresh thyme leaves)
- Season to taste with salt and pepper.
- Optional: serve with lemon wedges.

Directions:

1. Preheat the oven to 400°F (200°C). Line a baking sheet with parchment or aluminum foil.
2. In a large mixing bowl, mix together the Brussels sprouts, olive oil, chopped garlic, dried thyme, salt, and pepper. Toss the Brussels sprouts until they are equally coated.
3. Arrange the Brussels sprouts in a single layer on the prepared baking sheet, cut side down.
4. Roast the Brussels sprouts in a preheated oven for 20–25 minutes, or until soft and caramelized, tossing halfway through.
5. Once the Brussels sprouts have been roasted to your desired crispiness, remove them from the oven.
6. Transfer the roasted Brussels sprouts to a serving dish and, if preferred, garnish with fresh lemon juice.
7. Serve hot as a side dish or appetizer.

Tips

- To trim Brussels sprouts, take off rough ends and remove yellowing outer leaves before splitting lengthwise.
- Spread the Brussels sprouts in a single layer on the baking pan to promote uniform roasting and avoid overcrowding.
- Before serving, sprinkle the roasted Brussels sprouts with grated Parmesan cheese or balsamic vinegar for extra flavor.

- Leftover roasted Brussels sprouts may be refrigerated in an airtight container for up to three days. Heat gently in the oven or microwave before serving.

Health Benefits for Fatty Liver:

- Brussels sprouts are high in antioxidants, such as vitamin C and E, which help protect liver cells from inflammation and oxidative stress produced by fatty liver disease.
- Brussels sprouts' fiber content promotes good digestion and may aid in cholesterol regulation, which is useful for those with fatty liver disease.
- Garlic contains sulfur compounds that stimulate liver detoxification and enzyme synthesis, aiding in the treatment of fatty liver disease.
- The olive oil used in this dish contains beneficial monounsaturated fats, which have anti-inflammatory qualities and may help prevent liver fat formation when ingested as part of a balanced diet.

Quinoa Pilaf

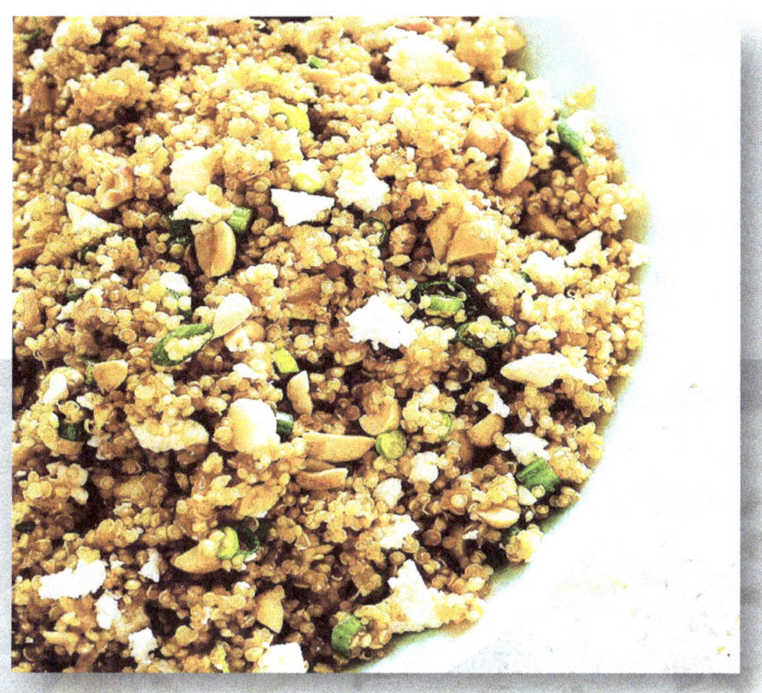

Preparation time: 10 minutes

Cooking time: 20 minutes

Total time: 30 minutes

Serving size: 4

Nutritional Data (Per Serving):

- Calories: 200 kcal.
- Six grams of protein.
- Fat: 8g
- Carbohydrate: 30 grams
- Fiber: 4 grams.

- Sugar: 2 grams.

- Sodium: 300 mg.

Ingredients:

- To prepare, combine 1 cup rinsed quinoa, 2 cups vegetable broth (or water), 1 tablespoon olive oil, 1 finely chopped onion, 2 minced garlic cloves, and 1 diced carrot.
- One chopped bell pepper.
- To prepare, add 1/4 cup chopped parsley, salt and pepper to taste, and optional lemon zest for garnish.

Directions:

1. In a medium saucepan, heat the vegetable broth to a boil. Add the quinoa, decrease the heat to low, cover, and cook for 15-20 minutes, or until the quinoa is tender and the liquid is absorbed. Remove from heat and allow to settle for 5 minutes before fluffing with a fork.

2. While the quinoa cooks, heat the olive oil in a pan over medium heat. Sauté the chopped onion until transparent, approximately 3–4 minutes. Add the minced garlic and simmer for another minute.

3. Add the chopped carrot and bell pepper to the pan and cook for 5–6 minutes, or until cooked.

4. When the quinoa is done, add it to the pan with the sautéed veggies. Add the chopped parsley, and season to taste with salt and pepper.

5. Serve the quinoa pilaf hot, topped with lemon zest if preferred.

Tip:

- Add other veggies like peas, corn, or spinach to personalize the quinoa pilaf.
- Spices such as cumin, paprika, or curry powder may be used to season the quinoa pilaf.
- Leftover quinoa pilaf may be refrigerated in an airtight jar for up to three days.

- Reheat gently in the microwave or on the stovetop before serving.

Health Benefits for Fatty Liver:

- Quinoa is a complete grain high in fiber, protein, and important minerals like iron and magnesium. Its high fiber content regulates blood sugar levels and
- Promotes digestion, which is useful for those suffering from fatty liver disease. Vegetables such as carrots and bell peppers include vitamins, minerals, and antioxidants that promote liver function and decrease inflammation.
- The olive oil used in this dish contains beneficial monounsaturated fats, which have anti-inflammatory qualities and may help prevent liver fat formation when ingested as part of a balanced diet.

Steamed asparagus with lemon butter

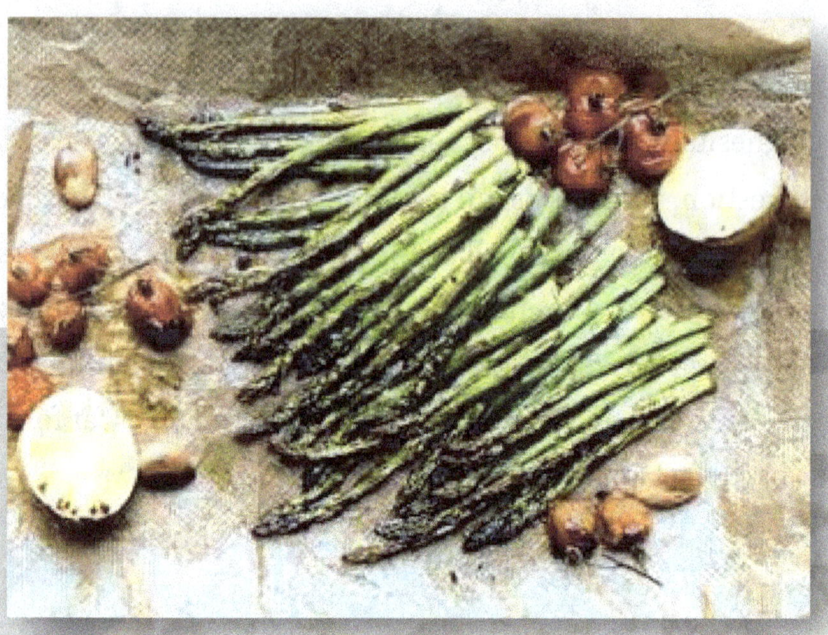

Preparation time: 5 minutes

Cooking time: 5 minutes

Total time: 10 minutes

Serving size: 4

Nutritional Data (Per Serving):

- Calories: 80 kcal.
- 3 grams of protein.
- Fat: 6g
- carbs: 6g
- Fiber: 3 grams.
- Sugar: 2 grams.
- Sodium: 150 mg.

Ingredients:

- 1 bunch asparagus, clipped ends, 2 tablespoons unsalted butter (or olive oil), and
- 1 tablespoon fresh lemon juice.
- Garnish with lemon zest
- Add salt and pepper to taste.

Directions:

1. Fill a big skillet or saucepan with approximately one inch of water. Put a steamer basket in the skillet and bring the water to a boil over medium-high heat.
2. Place the trimmed asparagus in the steamer basket, cover, and steam for 3 to 5 minutes, or until tender but still crisp.
3. While the asparagus steams, melt the butter in a small saucepan over low heat. Add the fresh lemon juice, and season to taste with salt and pepper.
4. Once the asparagus is done, place it on a serving tray and sprinkle with lemon butter sauce.
5. Garnish with lemon zest and serve immediately.

Tips:

- Avoid overcooking asparagus, which may turn mushy and lose its vivid green color.
- Grilling or roasting asparagus instead of steaming it will result in a distinct taste profile.
- Refrigerate any leftover steamed asparagus in an airtight container for up to three days. Reheat gently in the microwave, or serve cold in salads or sandwiches.

Health Benefits for Fatty Liver:

- Asparagus is a nutrient-dense vegetable rich in fiber, vitamins (including vitamin K, folate, and vitamin A), and antioxidants. Its natural diuretic characteristics may help alleviate fluid retention and bloating caused by fatty liver disease.

- Lemon juice contains vitamin C, an antioxidant that improves immunological function and protects liver cells from oxidative stress.
- The olive oil used in the lemon butter sauce contains heart-healthy monounsaturated fats, which may help decrease inflammation and enhance liver function when used moderately.

Mashed Cauliflower

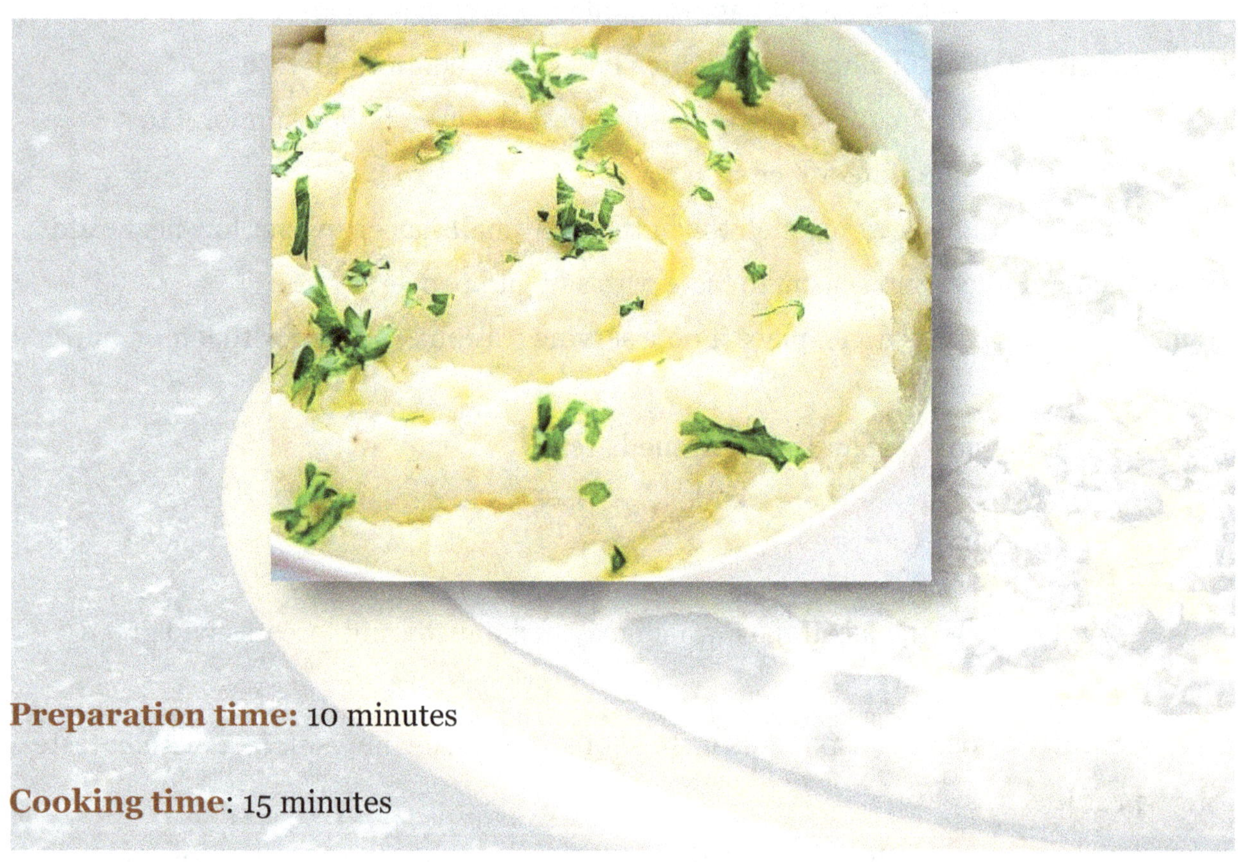

Preparation time: 10 minutes

Cooking time: 15 minutes

Total time: 25 minutes

Serving size: 4

Nutritional Data (Per Serving):

- Calories: 70 kcal.
- 3 grams of protein.
- Fat: 4g

- Carbohydrate: 7g
- Fiber: 3 grams.
- Sugar: 3 grams.

    Sodium: 200 mg.

Ingredients:

- One big head of cauliflower, chopped into florets.
- 2 garlic cloves, peeled
- 2 tablespoons unsalted butter (or olive oil)
- 1/4 cup grated Parmesan cheese (optional)
- Season to taste with salt and pepper. Garnish with chopped fresh herbs (optional).

Directions:

1. Heat a big saucepan of salted water to a boil. Cook the cauliflower florets and garlic cloves in the saucepan for 10–12 minutes, or until fork-tender.

2. Drain the cooked cauliflower and garlic, then place them in a food processor or blender.

3. To the cauliflower mixture, add butter (or olive oil) and grated Parmesan cheese (if desired).

4. Blend until smooth and creamy, scraping down the sides of the bowl as necessary. If the mixture is too thick, add a splash of milk or vegetable broth to get the correct consistency.

5. Season with salt and pepper to taste, then mix again until well incorporated.

6. Place the mashed cauliflower in a serving dish and garnish with chopped fresh herbs, if preferred.

7. Serve hot for a tasty and healthy alternative to typical mashed potatoes.

Tip:

- To enhance taste, toast cauliflower florets and garlic cloves before mashing.
  Feel free to season the mashed cauliflower with seasonings such as garlic powder,
  onion powder, or smoky paprika.
- Store leftover mashed cauliflower in an airtight jar in the refrigerator for up to
  three days. Reheat gently in the microwave or on the stovetop before serving.

Health Benefits for Fatty Liver:

- Cauliflower is a cruciferous vegetable that has a lot of fiber, vitamins (including
  vitamin C, vitamin K, and folate), and antioxidants. Its components may aid
  inliver detoxification and lessen the inflammation associated with fatty liver
  disease.
- Garlic contains sulfur compounds that aid liver function and stimulate enzyme
  synthesis in detoxification processes.
- The olive oil used in this dish contains heart-healthy monounsaturated fats,
  which may help decrease inflammation and enhance liver function when used in
  moderation.

Roasted sweet potatoes with rosemary

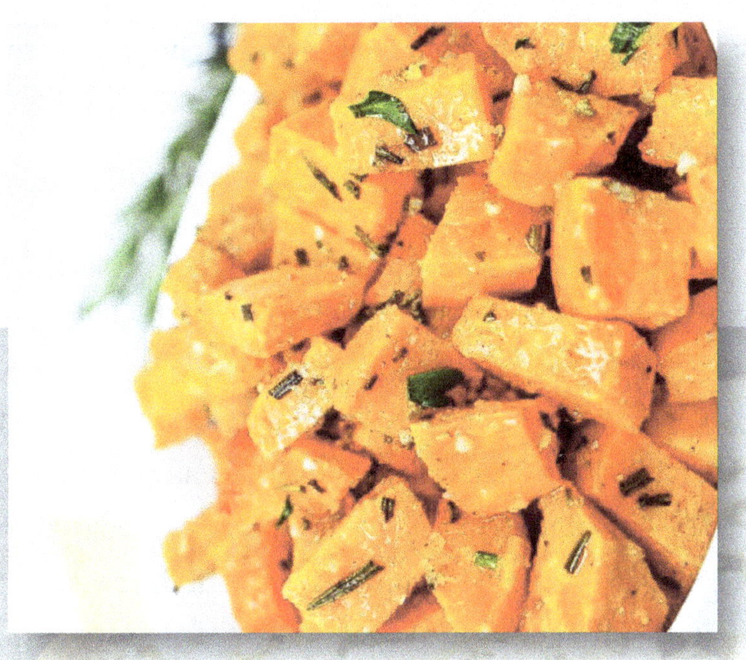

Preparation Time: 10 minutes

Cooking Time: 30 minutes

Total time: 40 minutes

Serving size: 4

Nutritional Data (Per Serving)

- Calories: 150 kcal.

- Two grams of protein.

- Fat: 4g

- Carbohydrate: 28 grams

- Fiber: 4 grams.

- Sugar: 8 grams.

- Sodium: 200 mg.

Ingredients:

- 2 big sweet potatoes peeled and cubed.
  Ingredients: 2 tablespoons olive oil, 2 tablespoons chopped fresh rosemary, and 2 cloves minced garlic.
  Add salt and pepper to taste.

Directions:

1. Preheat the oven to 400°F (200°C). Line a baking sheet with parchment or aluminum foil.
2. In a large mixing bowl, combine the cubed sweet potatoes, olive oil, chopped rosemary leaves, minced garlic, salt, and pepper until equally covered.
3. Place the seasoned sweet potatoes in a single layer on the prepared baking sheet.
4. Roast in the preheated oven for 25–30 minutes, or until the sweet potatoes are soft and caramelized. Halfway through, stir.
5. Once the sweet potatoes have been cooked to your desired crispiness, remove them from the oven.
6. Place the roasted sweet potatoes on a serving dish and, if wanted, top with more chopped rosemary leaves.
7. Serve hot as a tasty and healthy side dish.

Tip:

- For consistent cooking, keep sweet potato cubes comparable in size.
  To add more flavors, season with spices like paprika, cumin, or cinnamon.
- Leftover roasted sweet potatoes may be refrigerated in an airtight container for up to three days. Heat gently in the oven or microwave before serving.

Health Benefits for Fatty Liver:

- Sweet potatoes are high in vitamins (A, C, and B6), fiber, and antioxidants, which promote liver health and prevent inflammation linked with fatty liver disease.

- The olive oil used in this dish contains heart-healthy monounsaturated fats, which may lower inflammation and enhance liver function when used in moderation.
- Rosemary contains antioxidants and anti-inflammatory chemicals, which may protect liver cells from oxidative stress and improve overall liver function.
- Sweet potatoes' fiber content promotes good digestion and may aid in blood sugar regulation, which is useful for those with fatty liver disease.

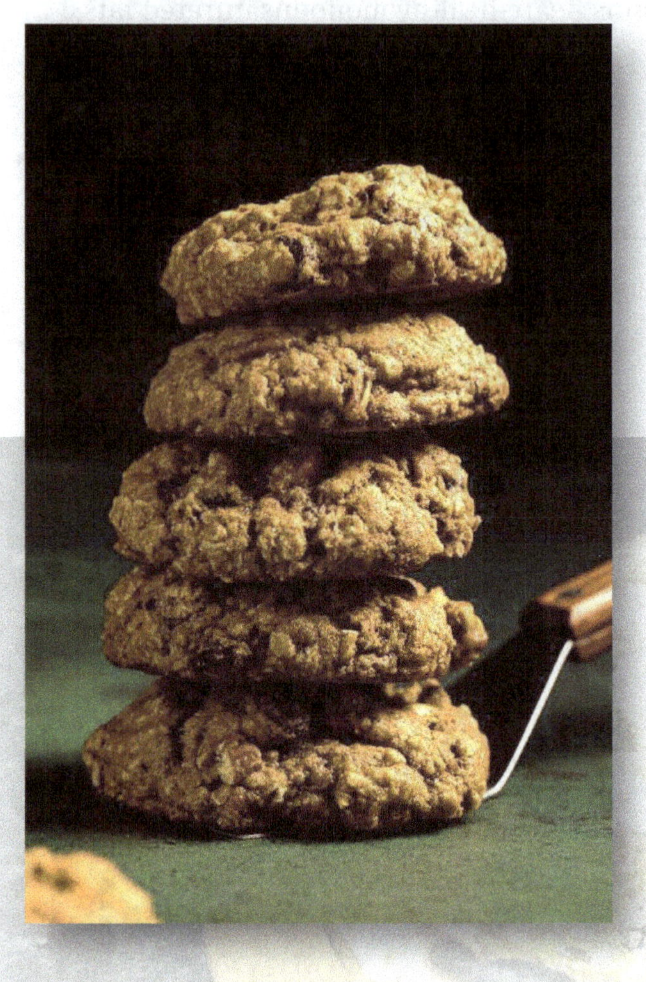

CHAPTER 6

DESSERTS

Desserts are delectable desserts served at the end of a meal, providing a sweet conclusion to culinary experiences. Desserts come in a variety of flavors, textures, and presentations to suit a wide range of tastes and preferences. Desserts, whether rich chocolate masterpieces, creamy custards, or the simplicity of fresh fruit, allow you to fulfill cravings while also celebrating special events. Desserts are frequently linked with indulgence, but they may also be made with nutritional ingredients, providing a good combination of flavor and health benefits. Desserts, with originality and expertise, may enrich dining experiences, making a lasting impact and providing delight to people who consume them.

Berry Chia Seed Pudding

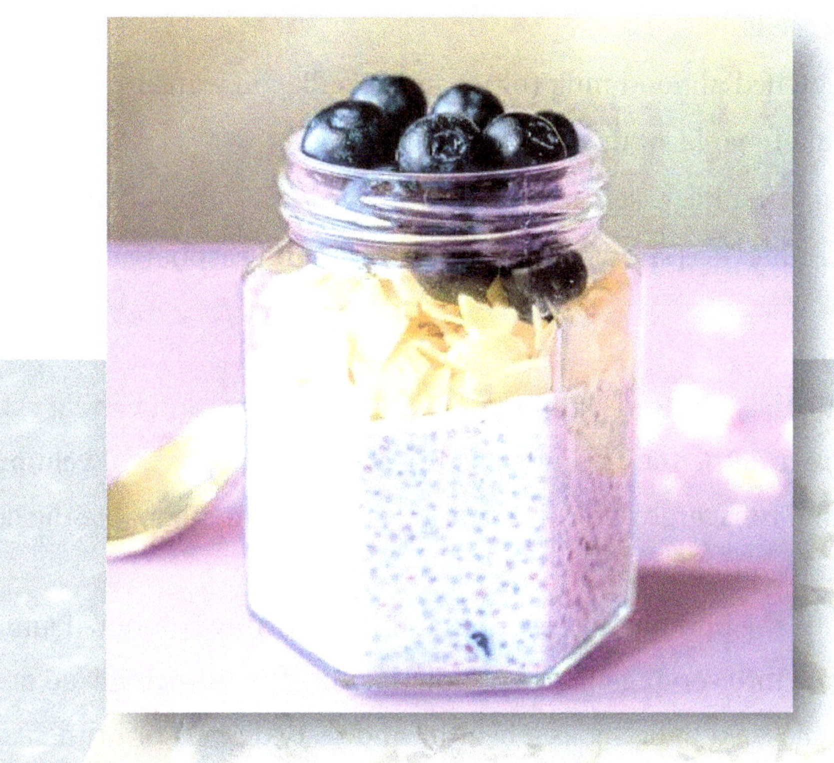

Prep Time: 5 minutes (plus overnight chilling)

Total Time: 5 minutes (plus overnight chilling)

Serving Size: 2

Nutritional Data (Per Serving):

- Calories: 150 kcal.
- 4 grams of protein
- Fat: 6g
- Carbohydrate: 20 grams
- Fiber: 8 grams.
- Sugar: 8 grams.
- Sodium: 50 mg.

Ingredients:

- 1/4 cup chia seeds.
- 1 cup unsweetened almond milk (or whatever milk you want)
- One spoonful of maple syrup (or honey)
- 1/2 teaspoon of vanilla essence.
- 1/2 cup mixed berries (strawberries, blueberries, and raspberries)

Directions:

1. In a dish, combine the chia seeds, almond milk, maple syrup, and vanilla extract.
2. Allow the mixture to settle for 5 minutes before stirring again to avoid clumping.
3. Cover the bowl and refrigerate overnight, or at least 4 hours, to enable the chia seeds to soak and thicken the liquid.
4. Before serving, stir the pudding to ensure that it is uniformly combined and smooth.
5. Spoon the pudding into serving glasses or bowls, and garnish with mixed berries.
6. Serve the berry chia seed pudding as a healthy and tasty dessert or brunch alternative.

Tips:

- Feel free to top the pudding with your favorite toppings, such as sliced bananas, chopped almonds, or coconut flakes.
- To adjust the sweetness level, add more or less maple syrup or honey according to your taste.
- Chia seeds are high in omega-3 fatty acids, fiber, and antioxidants, which promote heart health and may lower liver inflammation.

Dark Chocolate Avocado Mousse

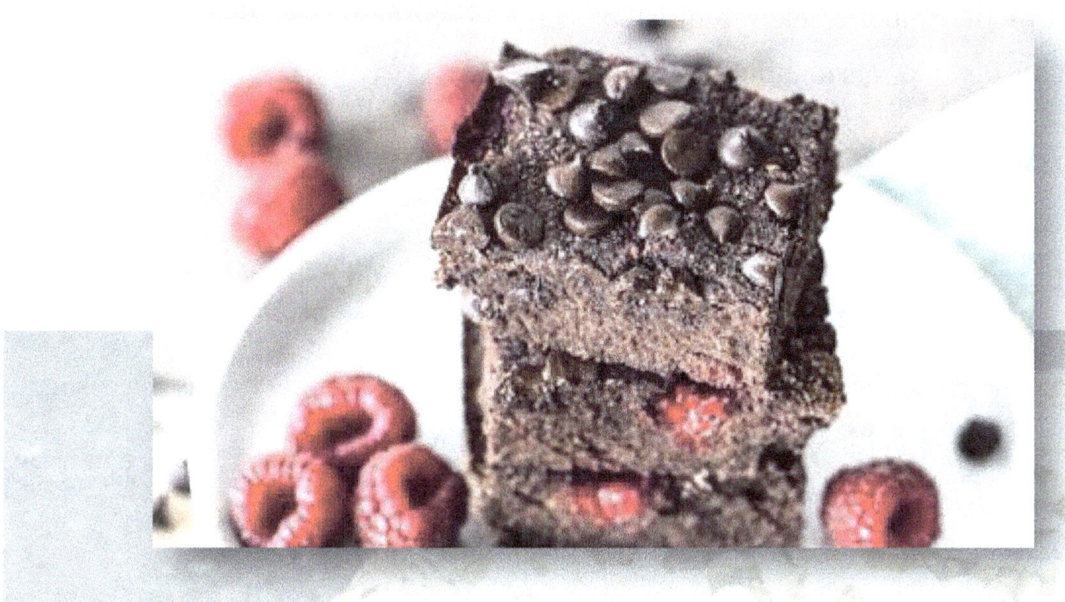

Prep Time: 10 minutes

Total Time: 10 minutes

Serving Size: 2

Nutritional Data (Per Serving):

- Calories: 200 kcal.
- 4 grams of protein
- Fat: 15g
- Carbohydrate: 15 grams
- Fiber: 6 grams.
- Sugar: 6 grams.
- Sodium: 10 mg.

Ingredients:

- One ripe avocado.

- Two teaspoons of cocoa powder.
- To make this recipe, combine 2 tablespoons maple syrup (or honey),
- 1/2 teaspoon vanilla essence, a pinch of salt, and optional fresh berries or shaved dark chocolate for garnishing.

Directions:

1. Scoop avocado flesh into a blender or food processor.

2. Combine the cocoa powder, maple syrup, vanilla essence, and a bit of salt in the blender.

3. Blend until smooth and creamy, scraping down the sides of the blender as necessary.

4. Taste the mousse and adjust the sweetness or cocoa flavor as needed.

5. Place the chocolate avocado mousse in serving glasses or bowls.

6. Optional garnishes include fresh berries or shaved dark chocolate.

7. Serve immediately, or chill until ready to serve.

Tip:

- Use ripe avocados for a creamy, smooth texture in the mousse.
- To give the mousse a deeper taste, mix it with a spoonful of nut butter or a splash of coconut milk.
- Avocados are high in monounsaturated fats, fiber, and antioxidants, all of which promote liver health and may help decrease inflammation caused by fatty liver disease.

Banana Oat Cookie

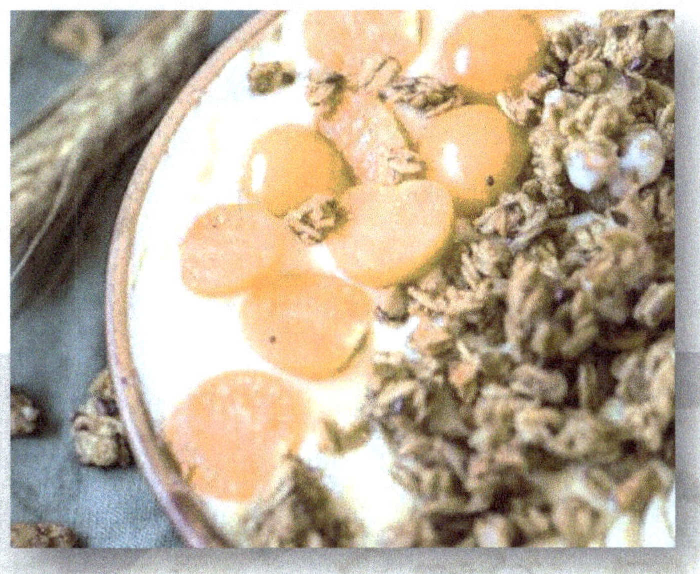

Prep Time: 10 minutes

Cooking Time: 15 minutes

Total Time: 25 minutes

Serving Size: 12 cookies

Nutritional information (per serving, one cookie):

- Calories: 100 kcal.
- Two grams of protein.
- Fat: 4g
- Carbohydrate: 15 grams
- Fiber: 2 grams.
- Sugar: 6 grams.
- Sodium: 30 mg.

Ingredients:

- Two ripe bananas, mashed
- One cup of rolled oats.
- 1/4 cup almond butter (or other nut butter)
- 1/4 cup chopped walnuts or chocolate chips (optional)
- One teaspoon of cinnamon.
- A pinch of salt.

Directions:

1. Preheat the oven to 350°F (180°C). Line a baking sheet with parchment paper.

2. In a mixing dish, add mashed bananas, rolled oats, almond butter, chopped almonds or chocolate chips, cinnamon, and a touch of salt. Stir until well blended.

3. Place spoonfuls of cookie dough on the prepared baking sheet, spreading them slightly apart.

4. Flatten each biscuit using the back of a spoon or fork.

5. Bake the cookies in the preheated oven for 15 minutes, or until golden brown and firm to the touch.

6. Remove the cookies from the oven and let them rest on the baking sheet for a few minutes before transferring them to a wire rack to finish cooling.

7. Try the banana oat cookies as a nutritious and enjoyable snack.

Tip:

- Customize cookies with dried fruit, coconut flakes, or seeds for added taste and texture.
- Leftover cookies may be stored in an airtight jar at room temperature for up to three days or frozen for longer.
- Bananas are high in potassium and fiber, which promote heart health and may help manage blood sugar levels, aiding those with fatty liver disease.

Baked Apples with Cinnamon

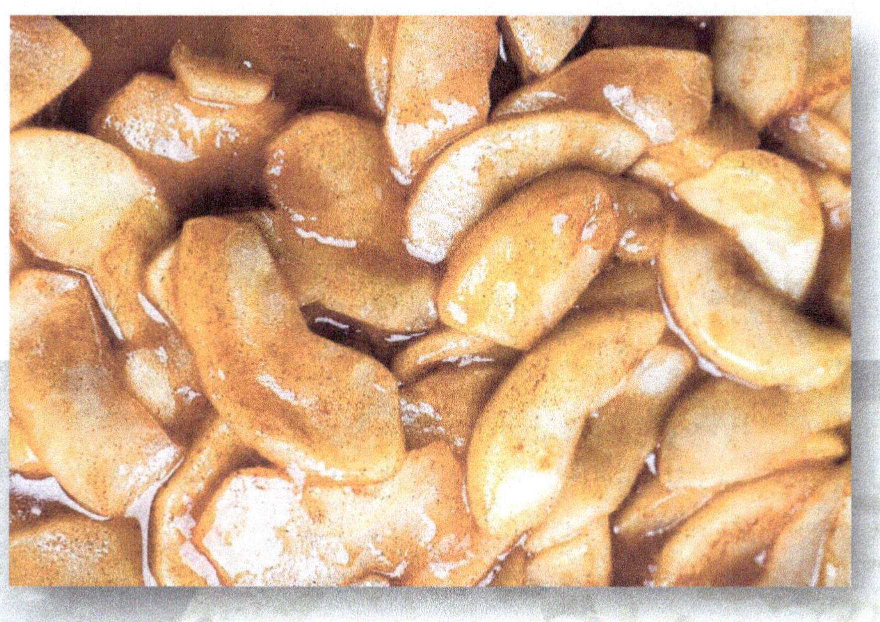

Prep Time: 10 minutes

Cooking Time: 30 minutes

Total Time: 40 minutes

Serving Size: 4

Nutritional Data (Per Serving):

- Calories: 120 kcal.
- Protein: 1g, fat: 0g.
- Carbohydrate: 30 grams
- Fiber: 5 grams.
- Sugar: 20 grams
- Sodium: 0 mg.

Ingredients:

- 4 medium apples (Granny Smith or Honeycrisp)

  two tablespoons of maple syrup (or honey).

- One teaspoon of ground cinnamon

- A pinch of nutmeg (optional).

- 1/4 cup of chopped nuts or dried fruit (optional).

Directions:

1. Preheat the oven to 375°F (190°C). Lightly grease or line a baking dish with parchment paper.

2. Core the apples using an apple corer or a knife, keeping the bottom intact.

3. In a small dish, combine the maple syrup, ground cinnamon, and nutmeg (if using).

4. Arrange the cored apples in the prepared baking dish.

5. Spoon the cinnamon mixture into each apple's center cavity.

6. If preferred, put chopped nuts or dried fruit on top of each apple.

7. Bake in a preheated oven for 25–30 minutes, or until the apples are soft and caramelized.

8. Remove the roasted apples from the oven and let them cool slightly before serving.

9. Serve the baked apples warm, either alone or with a dollop of Greek yogurt and a drizzle of honey.

Tips:

- Choose firm, somewhat sour apples.

- This recipe delivers the best results.

- Experiment with spices like cloves, ginger, and cardamom to enhance taste.

- Baked apples are a naturally sweet treat that is low in fat and calories, making them ideal for those with fatty liver disease.

DEAR VALUED CUSTOMER,

I hope you are enjoying your freshly acquired book!

I am glad that you chose to invest in my

Product and I appreciate you for that.

I recognize that your time is precious, and I am grateful for any further time you may be able to take to offer an honest evaluation. I feel that customer input is vital, and your opinions will help me produce an even better product in the future.

It would be very appreciated if you could take a few minutes to provide an honest review of this book. I genuinely respect your views and ideas and would be glad to get your suggestions on how I might improve.

I appreciate your devotion to my product, and I thank you for taking the time to offer an honest review.

Best Regard

ERNEST G. MOORE